THE SCIENCE AND ART OF
HAIR RESTORATION

PATRICK C. ANGELOS, M.D.

THE
SCIENCE
AND *Art* OF
HAIR RESTORATION

A PATIENT'S GUIDE

Advantage

Published by Advantage, Charleston, South Carolina.
Member of Advantage Media Group.

ADVANTAGE is a registered trademark, and the Advantage colophon is a trademark of Advantage Media Group, Inc.

Printed in the United States of America.

10 9 8 7 6 5 4 3 2 1

ISBN: 978-1-64225-127-2
LCCN: 2020906972

Book design by Megan Elger.

This publication is designed to provide accurate and authoritative information in regard to the subject matter covered. It is sold with the understanding that the publisher is not engaged in rendering legal, accounting, or other professional services. If legal advice or other expert assistance is required, the services of a competent professional person should be sought.

Advantage Media Group is proud to be a part of the Tree Neutral® program. Tree Neutral offsets the number of trees consumed in the production and printing of this book by taking proactive steps such as planting trees in direct proportion to the number of trees used to print books. To learn more about Tree Neutral, please visit **www.treeneutral.com**.

Advantage Media Group is a publisher of business, self-improvement, and professional development books and online learning. We help entrepreneurs, business leaders, and professionals share their Stories, Passion, and Knowledge to help others Learn & Grow. Do you have a manuscript or book idea that you would like us to consider for publishing? Please visit **advantagefamily.com** or call **1.866.775.1696**.

CONTENTS

ABOUT THE AUTHOR

DR. PATRICK ANGELOS is a facial plastic and reconstructive surgeon whose primary surgical interests include hair restoration and facial plastic surgery. He is certified by the American Board of Facial Plastic and Reconstructive Surgery and the American Board of Otolaryngology.

After graduating cum laude from the University of South Carolina Honors College, where he was selected as a Collegiate All-American Scholar, he then earned his medical degree from the Medical University of South Carolina. Dr. Angelos completed his residency at Oregon Health & Science University and was then selected for a prestigious fellowship in facial plastic surgery at the University of Illinois. In addition to various grants and awards, Dr. Angelos has been recognized as one of America's top surgeons since 2015.

Dr. Angelos's compassionate, thorough, and personalized approach has earned him a reputation as the area's trusted hair restoration and facial plastics expert. He combines his meticulous surgical skills with an artistic vision to achieve natural, lasting results.

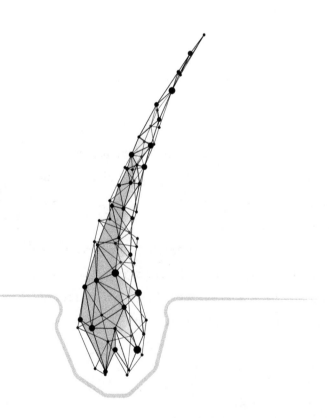

INTRODUCTION

With most patients that I see and treat, I haven't witnessed the actual progression of their hair loss. That wasn't the case with one of my earliest robotic hair restoration patients—my dad. Over the years, I had seen his hairline change, but he seemed to take it in stride, as if it was a natural part of aging. If he was bothered by it, he never let on—I never heard him talk about it making him feel older or less attractive. And I never heard him talk about trying any over-the-counter treatments. Then I began offering robotic treatment as part of the hair restoration services in my plastic surgery practice.

As an engineer, my dad was naturally curious about the new technology—he and I were both pretty intrigued to see how robotics could help reverse hair loss. After looking over the ARTAS System that I brought into my practice and getting a better understanding of how it worked, my dad expressed an interest in being one of my first patients.

While I was proud to get the chance to help my dad with his hair loss, I admit that I was a bit anxious. As a plastic surgeon, working on patients and helping them change their appearance was not new to me, and I had performed some minor cosmetic procedures on my dad in the past. But the robotics system was something new and different. And since hair transplantation is permanent, I knew we would be seeing my dad's results for the rest of his life.

When my dad came in for his first consult, he told me he had actually tried some different products to slow or stop his hair loss, but none of them had worked. He also hadn't found another hair restoration professional who made him feel confident enough to pursue other options. But he trusted me, so he was ready to see what the ARTAS System could do.

At age sixty-seven, he had pretty typical progression of hair loss around what's called the temporal recession areas, or those areas on top of the scalp above the eyebrows, along with some loss in the crown area, or the top of his head. His hair loss didn't really become noticeable until the hair on either side of his scalp was no longer connected to the hair on top. That gave him more of that "bald" look. On the Norwood Scale, he was a IV or V. The Norwood Scale classifies male pattern baldness on a scale of I through VII (one through seven), with Class VII being completely bald except for a ring of hair just above the ears and around the back of the head.

He, on the other hand, was most concerned about the prep before the procedure. On men, the procedure typically involves trimming existing hair very short, to about one millimeter. Basically, that's using an electric trimmer with no guard. It's a familiar concern for many men who pursue the ARTAS treatment. Sometimes, they comment, "I'm already worried about being bald, and I have to shave my head for this?"

Trimming the hair, however, gives us the best view of the hair and scalp and lets us take full advantage of all of the robot's features—its stereoscopic vision system, artificial intelligence, computer algorithm technology, and more.

The procedure takes some time to complete and made for a long day. But my dad was a great patient, and at the end of the day, like most patients, he was happy—and a little surprised—at how positive the transplantation experience was.

Using the ARTAS robotic hair restoration system, I was able to fill in the thinning areas and give him back a fuller head of hair. Today, we're both very happy with the results. Plus, he's receiving a lot of compliments from friends and family about how great he looks!

> Helping people obtain a more youthful look and feel better about themselves is why I became a plastic surgeon.

Helping people obtain a more youthful look and feel better about themselves is why I became a plastic surgeon. And it all started with a love of science and a talent for art.

A LOVE OF MEDICINE—AND ART

I've always been fascinated by biology and science. Growing up, I remember spending time at my grandmother's house looking through her books on plants and animals. Early on, I also had a talent for art. My mom and I used to do art projects together, and over time, art has continued to be a favorite hobby. Whenever I can, I like to paint and draw, take photographs, and even sculpt now and then.

As a youth, I was also involved in different sports activities, and by the time I was age fifteen, I had experienced about the same number of broken bones. My orthopedic surgeon was the father of one of my best friends, and it seemed like I was in and out of his office all the time getting a bone reset and placed in a cast. I also spent a lot of time being seen by my pediatrician for all the typical childhood ailments, and was in and out of my ear, nose, and throat (ENT) doctor's office for ear infections, tonsils, allergies, and a host of issues.

Yet I don't recall those experiences in a bad light. Instead, all that exposure to physicians growing up added to my decision to be a doctor. I always had a high respect for the doctors who treated me and was amazed at how fast they made me feel better.

After attending the University of South Carolina Honors College in Columbia, South Carolina, a university on par with Ivy League schools, I went to medical school at the Medical University of South Carolina in Charleston. Since I had so much exposure to orthopedic surgery as a youth, I naturally thought that was the path I would take. But after shadowing some orthopedic surgeons and seeing them do things like hammer knee implants into bone, which I viewed as more akin to carpentry-type work, I started to rethink.

I still wanted to be a surgeon and loved being in the operating room environment. But I wanted to see if there was a more artistic side to medicine, maybe one that involved finer details. That's when I discovered plastic surgery. I became especially interested in facial plastic surgery, which is a subspecialty of ENT.

To me, the anatomy of the head and neck are the most fascinating areas of the body because they are so complex—there are so many structures, including vessels, nerves, and bone, unlike other areas of the body. I decided to specialize in facial plastic surgery because it combined the complexity of the head and neck anatomy with the artistry of changing someone's appearance for reconstructive or cosmetic purposes. I headed to Portland's Oregon Health & Science University for a residency in otolaryngology, or ear, nose, and throat, and then I went to Chicago for a fellowship in facial plastic surgery.

In my practice today, I specialize in cosmetic and reconstructive surgery for areas involving only the head and neck. I also offer hair restoration, both medical and surgical options, in response to the growing desire for aesthetic treatments for men. While plastic surgery has long been something that primarily women sought out to change their appearance, in recent years we've seen a significant increase in men also looking for options—including hair restoration.

My practice, the Hair Restoration Center at Charleston Plastic Surgery, was the first in the state to offer state-of-the-art robotic restoration using the ARTAS System. We brought the system in after receiving many inquiries and realizing there was no one else in the area that we felt comfortable referring patients to. It's been a welcome addition to our hair restoration tool kit, giving patients some life-changing results.

MAKING A DIFFERENCE

When patients come to see me for an initial consult, it's usually pretty apparent that they are struggling with their appearance. But at the end of treatment, it's a different story—one of the most rewarding things about what I do is to see the positive impact on patients' confidence.

One of the challenges with hair restoration is that people put off treatment because of all the misinformation about their options. They're just not sure what really works, and no one wants to end up with "doll's hair," those little plugs that just don't look like natural hair. That's why I wrote this book. I want to inform you about hair loss in general, but I also want to share with you where we are with restorative treatments. There are many options for all kinds of hair loss in both men and women, and they work—they work very well.

Today's hair restorations are very natural looking, and the treatment is not terribly rigorous. Throughout the book, I will help clear up some of the myths to help you better understand that the options we have now are not, well, your grandpa's hair restoration.

Whether you're a man in your twenties and just beginning to notice some thinning, or you're in your sixties and experiencing advanced hair loss, you will find the information in this book useful in understanding medical and surgical options available today. There is also a chapter for women. While middle-aged women sometimes have noticeably thinning hair in the front, older women are often looking for solutions for diffuse thinning. The chapter explains some of the unique causes of hair loss in women, along with some treatment options.

I love what I do. I love seeing some of the exciting, life-changing results there are available today in hair restoration.

Let me tell you all about it.

CHAPTER 1

HAIR LOSS AND RESTORATION—
THE SCIENCE AND ART

*I*t happens to many of us. We look in the mirror one day and realize that we're starting to look a little different, a little older. In my practice, I see that happening to people at a younger age than you might think. When it comes to hair loss, guys as early as their thirties and forties, sometimes even in their twenties, see a change in their hairline that makes then cringe a little when they look in the mirror. Only yesterday, it seems, they had a full head of hair. What happened?

Sometimes, concern over hair loss really begins to take center stage when there's a life change or a big event around the corner. A wedding or divorce, new job or promotion, anniversary or reunion. Whatever the reason, it triggers or intensifies a nagging feeling that the person in the mirror is starting to look a little older—a little more like dad or granddad. Hair loss can cause or compound feelings of insecurity just when you want to look and feel your best. The same goes for women who experience hair loss.

One of the more subtle reasons that hair loss in the front is so disturbing is that it actually changes the framing of the face. The features of your face—your hair, ears, chin, and jawline—create a framework for that face you've seen in the mirror for years. When your hair begins to recede, it draws your hairline farther away from your eyes and makes your forehead appear larger. The whole portrait of your face changes because the top part becomes distorted. That can create an aging effect that can impact self-esteem in many people.

Yet, most of the time, when we see someone for an initial consultation, they have been thinking about treatment for a while. But they've put off seeking treatment for a variety of reasons. Some have finally reached a point where they can take off work for the treatment, or they finally have the means to feel comfortable about having something done.

Many have put off treatment simply because they are confused about their options. They've seen advertisements touting miracle restorative cures that, according to multiple online reviews or others they know that have tried the treatment, ultimately just don't work. Or they're sure they're going to end up with an unnatural result—it's common today to still equate hair transplantation with the "doll's hair" look that often resulted from treatment in the past. There is a lot of misinformation out there on what hair restoration is all about, but I'm going to share information to help clarify what hair loss and restoration is all about today. Treatments today produce natural-looking results that are nothing like hair restoration of the past.

THE TRUTH ABOUT HAIR RESTORATION

MYTH: Hair restoration is a painful process that results in a "doll's hair" look.

TRUTH: The ARTAS robotics system is not your grand-dad's hair restoration. It's a far more comfortable procedure that produces natural-looking results.

The truth is that there are both scientific and artistic components to hair loss and restoration. Let me first explain some of the basic science behind what causes us to lose hair.

HAIR LOSS SCIENCE—THE BASICS

When it comes to hair restoration, the majority of patients I treat are men who have experienced what is known as androgenic alopecia, what is commonly referred to as male pattern baldness but is also known as alopecia prematura, common baldness, and androgenetic alopecia. In the next chapter, I will discuss the differential diagnoses, or some of the most common causes of hair loss in men and women, but since male pattern baldness is so common, let me start there with some of the science.

The main driver of male pattern baldness is an excess of a hormone in the body known as dihydrotestosterone, what you may have heard referred to as DHT. DHT is actually created from testosterone through a conversion process involving an enzyme in the body.

Over time, too much DHT can cause hair to thin out—the strands themselves actually get smaller and smaller as the follicle shrinks from the effects of DHT. The follicle is the bulblike root of each strand of hair. Think of it like a perennial flower—you plant the bulb of the flower in the soil, and it grows back every year. Hairs go through a similar cycle. The follicle, that little bulblike root, lives in the scalp and draws blood supply and nutrients from the body. Every hair goes through a three-phase cycle: first growing, then transitioning, then resting. All hair is going through this same cycle, but at different times. Hairs can cycle indefinitely—longer than most of us live—but the effects of genetics, hormones, age, stress, and other factors can significantly shorten the number of cycles and how many hairs grow in each follicular unit. As the cycles decrease, the follicles shrink, and the strands of hair become thinner and thinner, turning into very fine, baby-type hair—peach fuzz, if you will—until they stop growing altogether. That's the progression of baldness.

Hair Growth Cycle

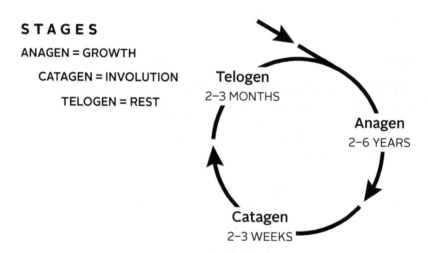

STAGES

ANAGEN = GROWTH

CATAGEN = INVOLUTION

TELOGEN = REST

Telogen
2–3 MONTHS

Anagen
2–6 YEARS

Catagen
2–3 WEEKS

Generally speaking, most, if not all of the medical treatments for hair loss are designed to help those miniaturized baby hairs turn back into more normal, full-size hairs. That gives the appearance of having more natural density in areas that previously appeared bald, helping to slow or even reverse the thinning process.

Once the follicles are gone, however, the only way to get more strands of hair in an area of thinning is to surgically transplant them back in by taking them from the scalp on the back and sides of the head. The hairs that grow in these areas are resistant to DHT.

There are three main steps to a hair transplant procedure. They involve three terms that I will use throughout the book: harvesting, site-making, and implantation.

- **Harvesting** is the actual removal of hair follicles from the back and sides of the scalp.

- **Site-making** is the act of preparing sites in other areas of the scalp (typically in front or on top) to accept the harvested hair follicles.

- **Implantation** is physically implanting the hair follicle grafts into the scalp.

While the concept of hair transplantation has been around for some time, the process itself has changed over the years, which has led to some dramatic improvements in results.

Hair transplantation's origins date back to wartime, when Japanese doctors noticed that the hairs in hair-bearing skin grafted to a burn victim's scalp would continue to grow. But those treatments were essentially forgotten after the war. Years later, a technique known as "punch grafting" was being used. It created the unnatural "doll's hair" look that people still equate to hair transplantation. Then, a technique known as "micrografting" was used, and it transitioned into a technique that uses more grafts with fewer hairs per graft to create a more natural look. I will share more details about the evolution of transplantation and bring us up to date with where we are now in chapter 4.

Today we know that transplantation works through what's known as the principle of donor dominance, which was discovered by Dr. Norman Orentreich. Donor dominance is the concept that hairs harvested from the back of the scalp and transplanted to the top will grow and remain there permanently. In fact, that's one of the best features of hair transplantation—and is why the art aspect of hair restoration is so crucial.

HAIR RESTORATION— THERE'S AN ART TO IT

It's often said that the good and bad of hair transplantation is that it's permanent. The good is that hair transplanted from the back of the scalp will become a permanent fixture wherever it is implanted— it will typically resolve any thinness or baldness you may have for the life. The bad, of course, is that if a hair transplant results in a hairline that really is not the best fit for your face, then it's still going to be permanent— it's going to be your new hairline now and forever.

> It's often said that the good and bad of hair transplantation is that it's permanent.

That's why the art of hair restoration is so important.

Researchers, over time, have developed a number of classification systems that give us some basic guidelines for restoring hair. One of the most widely used is the Norwood Scale, which identifies seven classes of hair loss in men from no hair loss to complete hair loss. There is also a classification system developed by Ebling, which looks at balding in Latin, Jewish/Arabic, and Nordic ethnic groups.[1] In Latin men, according to Ebling, recession begins at the front of the hairline, followed by thinning in the crown (also known as the vertex). Finally, those two areas blend together to form what is essentially a Class V on the Norwood Scale. In Jewish/Arabic populations, baldness moves from front to back until there is no hair remaining on the top of the scalp. Thinning in these men doesn't seem to occur as much in the crown as it does in Caucasians. Balding in men with a Nordic heritage, meanwhile, starts with a patch at the back of the scalp that progresses to the temple areas and may even leave an island of hair at the top that eventually disappears as well.

Research and various surveys also show that men in the Mediterranean area, particularly in Greece, Macedonia, and the Czech Republic, have the highest degrees of hair loss and balding, with more than 40 percent of men experiencing significant baldness. Japanese and East Asian men appear to have the lowest rates of hair loss, with any hair loss occurring later in life than in men in some countries, typically in their forties and fifties.

While the classifications are good starter guidelines, everyone's hairline is different, and every treatment is custom tailored. For example, if someone younger needs just a small amount of grafting at the front of the hairline or the temporal recession areas, then we don't want to exhaust all of their donor area. We also don't want to fill in the thinning area too much in case there is more progression later. If the crown is filled in and hair loss continues to progress around it, then you can end up with an island of transplanted hair—an unnatural result that could be compounded if no more donor hair is available for further transplantation.

---

1   Gustavo Gomez, *Hair Loss: Options for Restoration & Reversal*, (San Antonio: Halo Publishing, 2017).

Advising patients what's going to give them a good result now but still preserve the opportunity for doing transplantation later as the hair loss progresses is part of the art of hair restoration.

You see, male pattern baldness or hair loss is progressive and will continue until it reaches its end point. While we can estimate the extent of hair loss you will experience, primarily based on family traits, there is currently no way of knowing exactly where your hair loss is going to end up.

That's why part of the art of hair restoration is figuring out what treatments to use that will work for you now—and in the future. In addition to ethnic factors that might need to be considered, the art of designing the hairline also includes looking at photos of family members—a father, grandfather, and siblings—and of you at a younger age. That can help determine the natural progression of hairline changes over time.

One of the pluses of hair transplanted from the back of the scalp is that it will have the same features as the hair at the implantation site, so it blends in very well. Although color can sometimes vary from front to back, hair is a similar thickness and texture, no matter where it lives on your scalp.

One of the most important pieces of the art discussion is that of creating the appropriate angle during site-making. Hair in the front of the scalp actually grows at a very acute angle, usually straight forward or sometimes downward, toward the eyebrows. Hair transplanted to grow at a straight-up or backward angle will appear very unnatural—and can even be a dead giveaway that a transplant has been done. During manual transplantation, it's important for the doctor to make the implantation sites and insert the graft at the appropriate angle so that it appears very natural as it grows. When there is no hair present at the site to serve as a guide, then there are some basic norms that apply to most patients. In some cases, the whirl or pinwheel pattern at the crown is mimicked—however, when that is absent, then it must also be recreated to look natural. The crown should not be an island of hairs standing straight up; it should lie flat, just like a natural crown. There is certainly some finesse on the part of the doctor when it comes to angling the hairs appropriately during a transplant—it can really make all the difference.

I'm biased, but I feel like plastic surgeons do a better job than some other physicians that perform hair restorations. Since hair transplantation does not require any specific credentialing, it has become an add-on procedure for other healthcare providers who are not schooled or skilled at procedural medicine—and whose practices do not involve artistically restoring any part of the body, something that plastic surgeons do every day.

Not every patient needs hair transplantation. Especially when it comes to younger patients, it may be best to start with other options. Since the reasons for hair loss vary from person to person and are unique to their circumstances, a good place to start is by determining the cause of hair loss in the first place. In the next chapter, we'll look at a number of reasons for hair loss, along with some preventive measures that may help slow or even prevent hair loss long term.

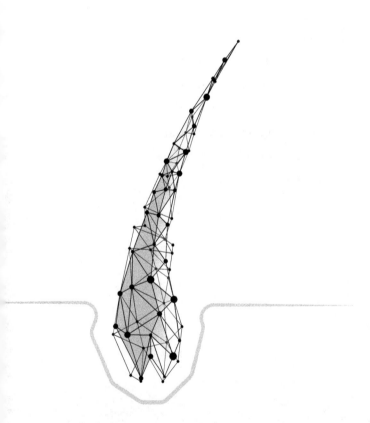

CHAPTER 2

WHAT CAUSES HAIR LOSS AND PREVENTIVE MEASURES

While it's normal to lose fifty to one hundred hairs per day, people I see in my practice often report losing an abnormal number of hairs. Over time, that leads to thinning and balding areas of the scalp. In South Carolina, where I practice, that's a problem for more than just aesthetics. It can leave the top of your scalp open to more than its share of the sun's rays. Men in this part of the United States are often not as concerned about their looks as they are about having to wear a hat in an area known for its sweltering heat.

So it's common for us to treat men experiencing androgenic alopecia or male pattern baldness due to genetics, hormones, and aging. In addition to looking more youthful and feeling better about themselves, they're looking for ways to protect their scalp.

But we also see men and women who are experiencing hair loss for a whole host of other reasons. Some have undergone a medical treatment, such as radiation or chemotherapy, that has led to hair loss on their scalp, eyebrows, and eyelashes. Some have a bare area on their scalp due to a trauma or a postcancer graft. Some are simply losing hair because they are currently under a lot of stress.

Whatever the reason for the hair loss, we look at each patient individually, first with a differential diagnosis, which is then finalized by further evaluation and testing as necessary, to determine the true cause (or causes) of that patient's hair loss. We want to get to the source of the problem before determining a solution, whether that's medical treatment or procedure, or transplant surgery.

Let's look at some of the causes of hair loss, and then I'll share preventive measures anyone can take to help deter hair loss in the first place. First, a little background.

HAIR LOSS—IT'S NOTHING NEW

Often, hair loss is thought of as a more modern condition because of factors such as stress, environment, and toxins in our world today. But the truth is that hair loss is nothing new.

In ancient Egypt, some physicians specialized in treatment of male pattern baldness, but without a lot of success in treating it. The ancient Greeks and Romans also had theories about hair loss. For instance, at one point, they suspected fumes of snake poison were culprits, and even the Greek physician Galen suspected "noxious elements" in the air contributed to hair loss. Hippocrates invented different topical concoctions to try to help with his balding scalp. He was one of the first to realize that baldness and testosterone were linked because he observed that castrated men did not lose their hair. Since they were not able to produce male sex hormones, they eventually did not have baldness.[2]

---

2   Gomez, *Hair Loss*, 53–55.

In the 1800s to early 1900s, one of the big theories was that hair loss was more prominent in people with oily scalps caused by a medical condition known as seborrheic dermatitis. To some degree, that is still true today. But even back then, people began to realize that medical or metabolic conditions like thyroid or iron deficiency could cause hair loss. They also began to realize that factors like stress and environmental conditions, such as radiation or smoke exposure, were also potentially playing a role in hair loss.

Today, we know that there are three factors in play when a man is experiencing male pattern baldness: genetics, hormones, and aging. Some of these may come into play with other types of hair loss, but in male pattern baldness, all three must be present. Other types of hair loss often come down to determining the differential diagnosis.

THREE MAIN FACTORS

If you're experiencing male pattern baldness, then you have a mix of three factors—genetics, hormones, and aging. If you have only one or two of these three factors going on, then you won't have male pattern baldness. Period. If you're experiencing hair loss, then we need to look a little further for the cause, and that will come with a diagnostic workup. For now, let's look at the three factors that lead to male pattern baldness and can cause hair loss in general.

Factor 1: Genetics

Historically, it's been believed that hair loss was passed down from the mother's side of the family, specifically from the maternal grand-father. In other words, whatever your mom's dad had in the way of a hairline, that's what you would end up with. As a child, I remember my parents and other adults saying, "Well, you probably won't go bald because your mom's dad has a pretty decent amount of hair." Even as research began to prove otherwise, that myth of inheriting the maternal grandfather's hairline was believed for a long time. While the hairline on that side of the family may certainly be a contributing factor, it's not the sole source. The hairline on both sides of the family typically plays into what you may inherit.

THE TRUTH ABOUT HAIR RESTORATION

MYTH: It's often believed that hair loss is passed down specifically from the mother's side.

TRUTH: Genetics from both sides of your family, along with hormonal and other factors, will determine your hairline.

There are actually multiple variations of a gene involved in hair loss (at least ten to thirty-five have been identified).[3] These gene variations are inherited primarily in an autosomal dominant fashion. This means that genetic predisposition is not sex linked and can come from either side of one's family. It's kind of like eye color. If you have traits for brown and potentially blue or green eyes, but brown is the dominant trait, then you're more likely to have brown eyes. Therefore, if balding genes are inherited, you will more likely than not have some degree of baldness.

Common baldness follows predictable patterns, as seen by the Norwood Scale.

---

3   "AR gene," *U.S. National Library of Medicine*, Genetics Home Reference, accessed February 10, 2020, https://ghr.nlm.nih.gov/gene/AR.

Norwood's Classification of Male Pattern Alopecia

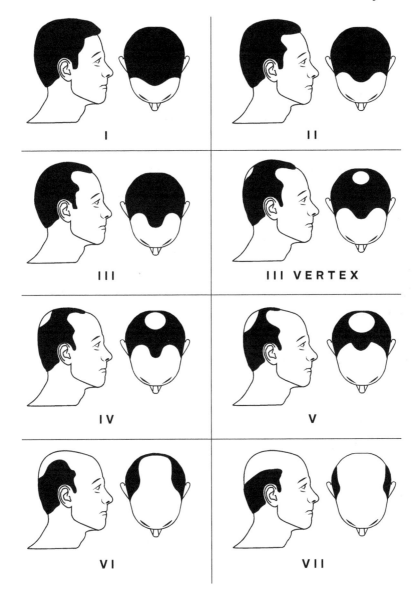

Even if you are genetically predisposed, however, you still must have the two other factors that I'm going to talk about—hormones and aging—for the genetic trait to manifest itself.

So even if you have baldness genes on both sides of the family, it's possible you will never become bald. It's also possible for baldness to skip a generation or two, even if the genes are present.

There's a variable expression of the genes that are related to hair loss. Gene expression is very basically understood as the instructions from our DNA as to how the gene should function (i.e., make proteins, signaling factors, and so forth) than manifest in a trait (hair loss). You may have genes that predispose you to hair loss, but the expression of those genes is what determines whether you will actually have hair loss. That varies based on innumerable factors, and it varies from person to person. Even if it appears you are predisposed to hair loss because of the hairlines on both sides of your family, your own genetics may not follow a prescribed path. No matter how strong the genetic predisposition, baldness will not happen if inciting agents such as steroids like testosterone and DHT are not present. On the contrary, if those agents are present but inherited genes for hair loss are not, then you won't go bald. In short, understanding the genetic factors that lead to hair loss is far more complicated than anyone originally thought.

> One thing we do know is that genetics, hormones, and aging are all interdependent.

One thing we do know, however, is that genetics, hormones, and aging are all interdependent.

Factor 2: Hormones

To explain how hormones impact hair loss, let me expand on some of the science I shared in chapter 1.

Androgens are basically any steroid hormone that stimulates the male sex organs or male sex characteristics. These are also termed anabolic steroids because of the way that they are converted by the body's biochemistry. Testosterone and DHT are considered androgens, and they have the biggest impact on hair loss and specifically male pattern baldness.

Testosterone gets converted into DHT by a specific enzyme known as 5-alpha-reductase. DHT specifically binds to receptors on hair follicle cells, causing the specific changes associated with balding. DHT slows down the growing phase of the hair cycle and causes miniaturization. Over time, the hairs get smaller and smaller until they turn into baby-type hair before they stop growing altogether and you lose follicles. However, the miniaturization process is not solely dependent on the steroid hormones. It's a slow process, which is why it's also dependent on aging. Some of the medications that I'll talk about in the next chapter block the conversion process of testosterone to DHT and help slow or even reverse miniaturization.

Certain areas of the scalp are more susceptible than others to the effects of DHT. For example, the sides and the back of the hair don't typically have hair loss because those hairs are more DHT resistant. That's actually how and why transplantation works—even though DHT levels may be present in the implant areas, the hair will still continue to grow just like it would on the sides and back because it's taken from DHT-resistant areas of the scalp.

Interestingly, the mostly illegal anabolic steroids that bodybuilders sometimes take to build muscle can actually cause hair loss. Men taking these supplements tend to lose hair because, by driving up testosterone levels, they're also driving up DHT levels. That's the opposite of what most people think—they're under the misconception that taking testosterone will build hair all over their body, but the truth is that it can cause hair loss. As I write this book, there are a lot of commercials advertising testosterone supplements for low T, low libido, low energy, and so on. Those may make you feel better, but it's very possible you will experience hair loss as a side effect. Some people try to offset the hair loss by taking a DHT-blocker like Propecia, but the combination of the two—rising testosterone levels, especially above normal, and taking Propecia—may actually increase overall hair loss.

THE TRUTH ABOUT HAIR RESTORATION

MYTH: Taking testosterone will cause more hair to grow all over the body.

TRUTH: Testosterone supplements can actually cause hair loss.

Human growth hormone (HGH), an anti-aging supplement that some people take to feel younger, can also cause hair loss. Fitness-focused individuals also sometimes take supplements that can potentially cause hair loss. These include whey-based nutritional supplements, DHEA, and supplemental steroids. I'm not talking about the short course of steroids that you might take for a medical condition such as a sinus infection or a flare-up of asthma. But long-term steroids, like Prednisone, taken for years for rheumatoid arthritis or other autoimmune diseases can certainly cause hair loss. I'll talk about this more in chapter six on hair loss in women.

Factor 3: Aging

Obviously, there is a link between aging and hair loss. Not only does it occur more commonly in people as they grow older, but it also tends to be more extensive when it starts at a younger age.

The bottom line is that most men who are going to have extensive balding develop a lot of it by age thirty. In fact, statistics show that a certain percentage of men will experience hair loss as follows:[4]

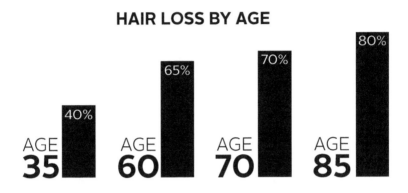

HAIR LOSS BY AGE

AGE 35 — 40%
AGE 60 — 65%
AGE 70 — 70%
AGE 85 — 80%

Aging hair tends to change in color, texture, and thickness. Apart from male pattern baldness, there is a unique condition known as senescent alopecia that is a very slow progression of diffuse hair loss. That condition may coexist with male pattern baldness in some men in their late fifties, sixties, and seventies. Other important factors associated with aging and hair loss include what are thought to be oxidative stress changes within the hair follicles that affect how they cycle over time.

Again, aging is interdependent with the other factors—genetics and hormones—to affect hair loss and cause it to slowly progress. And it's not a steady progression—hair loss rates can speed up, slow down, and even stabilize over time. However, it does seem to slow down a little bit by the time men reach their mid- to late sixties. Men who start losing their hair in their twenties will probably have more significant baldness than those who start the process in their thirties and forties.

---

4 Gomez, *Hair Loss*, appendix.

In addition to these three factors, there are other contributors to the big picture of hair loss.

STRESS

Stress is certainly a factor in hair loss because it can affect hormone levels. Loss of a child, layoff from a job, a family member diagnosed with a life-ending illness, or another major psychologically stressful event can cause a sudden loss of hair that will typically grow back over time. That's why we ask about life situations during the consult. We want to know whether you are experiencing extreme stress that has you completely overwhelmed. If we find that's the case, then rather than treating for male pattern baldness or other causes, we will likely recommend waiting to see whether the hair returns.

Stress is almost certainly a factor behind conditions, such as telogen effluvium, which is a reversible, rapid shedding of the hair during the resting phase (the telogen phase). It happens when the body senses a very stressful event and it needs to divert its energy away from growing hair.

There is also a stress-related medical condition, trichotillomania, which is basically a form of obsessive-compulsive disorder (OCD) where a person continually pulls or plucks their hair or scratches at their scalp, and that eventually causes hair loss that may not grow back with time. Regrowth depends on the level of scarring that is done to the scalp.

SCALP BLOOD SUPPLY AND CIRCULATION

DHT causes inflammatory damages to the circulation, and that can deprive hair follicles of blood and vital nutrients. But even though it appears that blood supply keeps follicles happy and healthy, there is still some controversy on whether diminished blood supply is actually responsible for hair loss.

A few Japanese studies have found that young men with male pattern baldness had more than two-and-a-half times lower scalp blood flow than in normal controls.[5] Other theories say that when there are no hair follicles in the area, some of the blood supply goes away. And we know bringing in new follicles can increase the blood supply. Other researchers, including some at Massachusetts General Hospital, have grown hair faster and thicker in mice that were given proteins that promote new blood vessel growth.[6] Research has also found that identifying and adding growth factors that stimulate blood vessel growth can help with hair follicle vascularization, promoting hair growth and increasing follicle size.

So does blood supply diminish after the hair is gone? Or is it the lack of blood supply that causes hair loss? Certainly, where there's more hair, there's more blood supply, and even when new grafts are transplanted into areas that don't have good blood supply, blood supply does increase. It's even been found that blood supply will increase in scars or skin grafts with no hair. These areas have been implanted with new follicles that survive, so scalp circulation changes are not fully understood.

---

5   William Cranwell, "Male Androgenetic Alopecia," *Endotext*, February 29, 2016, accessed August 5, 2019, on NCBI, https://www.ncbi.nlm.nih.gov/books/ NBK278957/.

6   Gomez, *Hair Loss*.

It's also theorized that muscle tightness in the scalp can potentially contribute to hair loss. This is especially common in people who have issues with dystonia (a muscle contraction disorder) and other conditions such as temporomandibular joint dysfunction. More commonly known as TMJ, this condition causes clenching and grinding of the teeth at night, which can lead to chronic tension in forehead and scalp muscles. The theory is that all that tension can contribute to hair loss, and that may relate to a decrease in blood flow and circulation. People have tried Botox treatments to relax the muscles in the scalp to see if that will help with hair loss, but I think this is an area that needs more research.

ENVIRONMENTAL FACTORS

While early theories looked at environmental factors like pollution and smoking as causes of hair loss, some recent studies are pointing to free radical damage as contributors. Free radicals are atoms in the body that can damage the DNA in your cells. Free radicals can be triggered by pollution, radiation, cigarette smoke, and maybe even herbicides. These environmental factors and free radical damage to DNA in hair stem cells and other hair follicle cells may impact hair growth and cycling. Although the role of environmental factors is likely small, further investigation into this area continues.

NONSCARRING AND SCARRING CONDITIONS

Some types of hair loss are caused by conditions that are either transient or leave more permanent scarring. The big distinction between the two is that with scarring of the follicles, hair loss in the area is often *irreversible*. These areas will not typically grow new hair with medical treatments alone.

During a consultation, we sometimes conduct a scalp biopsy to determine whether the condition is the scarring or nonscarring type of alopecia. That can help us see whether we need to take a wait-and-see approach, or whether their scalp may respond to medical treatments and reverse the process. If it's causing scarring, the hair is less likely to return, and transplant may be the only option. But if it's nonscarring, then with treatment, we're more likely to get the condition under control and improve the chances that the hair will come back.

Here is a brief differential diagnosis of nonscarring and scarring conditions that we see during consultations, with androgenic alopecia, again, being by far the most common balding condition.

Nonscarring Conditions

Alopecia areata. This is one of the more common nonscarring scalp conditions. It's an autoimmune disease that causes a patchy, circular-pattern hair loss. It's usually very easy to diagnose and treat.

Telogen effluvium. This is stress-related and causes rapid loss of hair. Again, normal shedding is about one hundred hairs a day. But losing four hundred or more hairs per day is not normal. That can happen at any age and may be a bit more common in women. It tends to fluctuate with hormone levels postpregnancy or postmenopause. Basically, it happens because it shifts all the hairs into a resting phase for a certain period, which is why it's reversible. The hair tends to come back after the body realizes that the stressful event is over.

Anagen effluvium. Anagen is the growth phase of the hair cycle.

Anagen effluvium is most commonly caused by chemotherapy drugs, which attack rapidly dividing cells like hair. Typically, the hair does come back over time, but it may change a little bit in color and texture and may be a little thinner or thicker in some areas.

Tinea capitis. This is basically a fungal infection of the scalp.

Thyroid conditions. Thyroid levels, especially hypo-, or low, thyroid levels, may affect metabolism on the hair follicles.

Anemia and iron deficiency anemia. This occurs when the blood lacks healthy red blood cells. Iron deficiency is a common cause of anemia.

Diabetes. The effects of diabetes can include endocrine or steroid imbalances, stress, and poor circulation.

Malnutrition. Conditions of malnutrition, as occurs with anorexia, can lead to significant hair loss, especially if there's deficiency of certain nutrients, vitamins, minerals, and elements required for healthy hair growth.

Psoriasis. This is a chronic skin condition indicated by patchy, red, scaly skin. It is caused by an overactive immune system. Areas of affected scalp may show temporary or permanent hair loss.

Syphilis. Hair loss may occur, especially in secondary or latent syphilis. Lab tests during consult to evaluate for an unknown cause of hair loss include a test for syphilis, primarily to rule it out.

Postpartum. This period or time frame can affect hormone levels in women and may be connected to telogen effluvium from a stressful event. The thought is that pregnancy hormones may increase the growing phase of the hair cycle, and then after pregnancy, there is a shift toward the other phases of the hair growth cycle, which includes the telogen phase. That can lead to more shedding after pregnancy. Thankfully, for new moms, this is usually temporary hair loss.

Trichotillomania. This is a form of OCD and involves self-damage to the hair and scalp. Regrowth depends on the level of scarring. Psychiatric help may be indicated for these patients who struggle to get this condition under control.

Traction alopecia. Probably the most common example of traction alopecia is wearing very tight braids, dreadlocks, or weaves. These constantly put tight traction on the follicles and can lead to hair loss that could be permanent. If caught early enough, traction alopecia can be nonscarring, but in its later stages, it can have some degree of scarring.

Scarring Conditions

Scarring is sometimes secondary to damage from other causes. In most cases, regrowth won't occur in scarred areas of the scalp with medical treatments alone. Transplantation may be the only option for restoration if the underlying condition can be stabilized medically.

Scarring conditions include:

- **Lichen planopilaris**, a skin disease that targets hair follicles.

- **Frontal fibrosing alopecia**, which leads to slowly progressive hair loss at the temples and front of the scalp.

- **Pseudopelade**, a kind of permanent loss that occurs in patches.

- **Dissecting cellulitis of the scalp**, which is similar to a bad, cystic acne kind of condition.

A Scarring and Nonscarring Condition

Lupus is an autoimmune disease that can cause both scarring and nonscarring types of alopecia. **Systemic lupus** typically causes nonscarring hair loss. **Discoid lupus** tends to be more localized, but it can cause a scarring type of hair loss.

MEDICATIONS

There are a number of medications that can also cause hair loss. These include:

- **Acne medications.** Medications for acne include isotretinoin or Accutane.

- **Anti-inflammatory drugs.** Nonsteroidal anti-inflammatories, or NSAIDS, can cause hair loss. These include the brand Naprosyn or the generic naproxen.

- **Antidepressant medications** like Paxil, Prozac, and Zoloft.

- **Beta-blockers.**

- **Birth control pills.**

- **Blood thinners**, including Coumadin, or the generic warfarin.

- **Gout medications**, including the generic allopurinol.

- **Seizure medications.**

- **Acid reflux medications** like Pepcid and Zantac.

- **Chemotherapy drugs.**

What I've shared with you are only some of the reasons that people experience hair loss. Again, most of the patients we see are dealing with androgenic alopecia, or male pattern baldness. For them, genetics, hormones, and aging are all factors that we need to consider when looking at solutions. But stress, blood supply and circulation, environmental factors, various scarring and nonscarring conditions as reviewed, and medications can all contribute to some degree of hair loss.

While the information I've shared is fairly comprehensive, understand that there may be many reasons why you're losing hair. For some people, it's a matter of changing habits or early intervention to prevent hair loss in the first place. It is most beneficial to take a comprehensive and individualized approach to hair restoration.

I had the procedure to help with my receding hairline. I can't speak to results yet, as I am only two months removed from having the procedure, but I would love to tell you how great the staff is ... they are all incredibly nice and knowledgeable. My procedure was painless and easy. They did everything possible to make me feel comfortable during my procedure. You can also tell they really care for their patients. I would 1,000 percent recommend Charleston HRC, Artas, and this staff! **—Z. L.**

PREVENTIVE MEASURES

Understanding your genetic risk is a big part of prevention. If your dad or older brothers have thinning hair, a receding hairline, or balding, then you may be at a genetic risk. Identifying and treating that early may help you have better results in preventing the progression of hair loss.

Along those same lines, if you think you may be at genetic risk, then evaluating and treating any hormonal issues or imbalances that might be affecting or accelerating hair loss may also help you early and in the long run.

Other ways to help prevent hair loss include:

Have good hair care and hygiene habits. When washing hair, massage your scalp, rinse well with cold water, and avoid pulling back on your hair because that can put traction on the follicles. The same goes for combing. It's less stressful on the follicles to wash and comb your hair forward, toward your face, instead of toward the back of your scalp and neck. Also, long hair weighs more, so on its own, it can put more traction on the follicles.

Regularly brushing hair, however, is actually good for it—brushing massages the scalp and helps improve blood flow and circulation. Brushing your hair once a day, especially with a brush that can stimulate the scalp, is almost as good as shampooing your hair. That's partly because brushing can help remove dirt from the scalp. It's also important to keep your combs and hairbrushes clean.

The condition of your hair should also be in balance—not too oily, not too dry. Also avoid overuse of a hair dryer on your hair—that can make it weak and brittle, which can lead to more hair loss.

Treat health issues. Treat any hormonal imbalances or other medical conditions such as low thyroid or iron or iodine deficiency, which can contribute to hair loss.

Avoid overuse of supplements and medications. Since supplements such as testosterone, HGH, whey, and DHEA can cause thinning and hair loss, avoid excessive use of these.

Watch your nutrition. Some fad diets may have a nutritional impact on hair loss. In my opinion, it's really important to eat a healthy balance of carbohydrates, proteins, and fat.

Also take a multivitamin that includes vitamins A, B complex, C, D, and E, along with the minerals zinc, iodine, and iron. You may want to also take a supplemental B-complex vitamin, although most multivitamins have sufficient amounts of Bs. And, if not in the multivitamin, also supplement with biotin, a coenzyme that helps the function of B-complex vitamins.

Avoid unhealthy environments. Avoid radiation exposure and air pollution that may be contributing to hair loss. More specifically, avoid smoking, not only because of its negative health effects but also because it can affect hair loss.

If you can identify some of the potential causes for hair loss that may not specifically be male pattern baldness, you may find successful treatment through a hair care professional, a dermatologist that specializes in scalp conditions, or a plastic surgeon or other hair transplant specialist who also treats these conditions.

In the next chapter, I'll talk about nonsurgical options, more specifically for male pattern baldness but which also can help other kinds of hair loss.

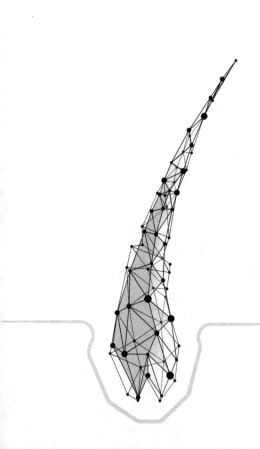

CHAPTER 3

NONSURGICAL TREATMENT OPTIONS

igs, hairpieces, extensions, spray-on thickening—
these are some of the solutions that people use for
thinning or balding hair. They may have already tried
some heavily touted remedy that didn't work and, fed
up, they just resorted to covering up or masking their missing hair.
In fact, without consulting a hair restoration professional, it's hard
to know whether a treatment may be interacting with something
else and even causing more hair loss. You may be trying to self-treat
what you believe is condition X with a solution that only works
for condition Y. Men, for instance, sometimes believe that they're
dealing with male pattern baldness, but their hair loss is really due
to some other cause. So the treatments that they're using may not
necessarily work.

Often, the patients we see are so frustrated with the solutions
they've tried that they think surgery is their only option. Sometimes,

those patients are in their twenties or thirties, and they just immediately want to do transplantation. But at that age, it may not be worth the cost and may even complicate transplantation later on. Sometimes, frustrated patients are in more advanced stages of hair loss, but for any number of reasons, they're just not ready to commit to surgery.

Whatever the case, patients often come in for a consult because they just don't realize that there may be other nonsurgical options available. Typically, we try to maximize medical treatments to see how much regrowth patients can get before we look at surgery. Medical treatments can help rebuild hair that is thinning and keep many patients happy for many years before transplantation becomes a better option.

MEDICAL OR PROCEDURAL TREATMENTS

If thinning and miniaturization are the issues, then maximizing some medical or procedural treatments may give really good results and preserve your hair for a long time. Medical and procedural treatments can slow down or stop hair loss. They can help miniaturized hairs gain back some volume by getting the small, baby hairs to turn back into more normal-sized hairs. However, these treatments don't help grow new follicles. That can only be done by transplantation.

Since hair loss is a progressive problem, you have to continue these treatments to stay ahead of the lifelong contributors of hormones, genetics, aging, and other factors.

Like all other medical treatments for hair loss, you really

have to commit to these for life. Since hair loss is a progressive problem, you have to continue these treatments to stay ahead of the lifelong contributors of hormones, genetics, aging, and other factors. Otherwise, you may lose any progress you've seen and even have further progression.

Here are some medical and procedural treatments that have proven effective.

Topical Treatments

Topical treatments are applied to the scalp only in the areas of hair loss. Some of these are more effective in younger patients who are going through the process of thinning. None of these are really as effective as you get more advanced loss.

Here are some of the topical treatments that are in use today. Which of these we prescribe depends on the situation.

Minoxidil. The most common brand name for minoxidil is Rogaine. When it initially came out, minoxidil was a blood pressure medicine. But doctors and patients observed that it not only helped with blood pressure, it also had a side effect of growing body hair. That led to its use on the scalp to get some regrowth of hair.

Minoxidil is a vasodilator, which means it helps increase blood flow to the scalp wherever it's applied, and that leads to some of that regrowth of the small hairs—it makes existing hairs stronger and thicker. It also increases the duration of the growth phase of the hair cycle. Basically, it shifts more of the hair into a growing phase and away from the resting phase. The results tend to be more hair growing for a longer period of time. And the hairs are thicker and less miniaturized.

Minoxidil really does work well for men and women, but it

tends to work better in the front of the scalp than on the crown. It's typically applied once or twice a day to the affected area. We typically advise only once a day, because it has a long half-life of about twenty-four hours. However, it should be applied only where you want hair to grow—you don't want it to get onto other areas of the scalp or face because it will create growth wherever it's applied. It is very well tolerated by most people with the most common side effects reportedly being redness, itching, scalp irritation, or unusual hair growth on other areas of the face. In a few rare cases, some people have reported headaches and dizziness.

The results can start to be seen in roughly six months. After a couple of years, the medication gradually becomes less effective. Still, like a lot of medical treatments, you must continue using it or you will experience some reversion. In fact, you will likely lose all the gains if you do not continue the treatment.

With minoxidil, there are different concentrations available. We generally recommend the 5 percent concentration for men and women. Some practices recommend only the 2 percent for women, since that is available over the counter. But in the state where I practice, the 5 percent is only available by prescription, so we provide it to patients through my practice or provide a prescription that they can fill at a pharmacy. It's available as an oil, lotion, or foam; of these, the foam seems be more tolerable and less irritating to most patients.

Retin-A or tretinoin. Retin-A is a vitamin A derivative that is a biological modifier. It can regulate some of the cell growth at the top layers of the skin and promote more blood vessel growth. Many transplant doctors and dermatologists who treat for hair restoration recommend a Retin-A topical along with minoxidil because the combination has been shown to triple the absorption rate of minoxidil.

The only side effect in some people is a little redness in the area where the treatments are applied.

Follicular therapy sprays or copper peptides. Some more common sprays or copper peptides used today are Tricomin and Folligen follicular sprays. There are also many OTC products that are hair follicle stimulators and "energizers." These may have some marginal effectiveness for now, but may be more of a mainstream treatment option in the future.

Oral Medications

There are a number of oral medications that are effective in preventing the progression of hair loss. Here are some that we prescribe, and others that are sometimes prescribed off-label.

Rogaine and Propecia are both FDA approved for hair loss, and are by far the most common treatments used.

> Rogaine and Propecia are both FDA approved for hair loss, and are by far the most common treatments used.

Finasteride. Finasteride is a medication that prevents the conversion of testosterone to DHT by blocking the 5-alpha reductase enzyme. Commonly known by the brand name Propecia, finasteride is by far one of the best oral medical treatments available for prevention of hair loss and for maintaining as much hair as possible. Propecia is a one milligram tablet taken once a day.

Proscar is another brand of finasteride that is commonly prescribed for a prostate condition, benign prostatic hyperplasia (BPH). Although it's prescribed for BPH, patients that take it may experience hair maintenance benefits. It is taken in a five-milligram daily dose.

Some of the side effects of finasteride make it a less-popular option for some people. Specifically, there are some sexual side effects that can be long term for a very small percentage of patients, even after stopping the medication. This is a condition known as post-finasteride syndrome.

Still, we often recommend finasteride because it can be extremely effective at lowering DHT levels and really have an effect on preventing the progression of hair loss over time.

Dutasteride. Commonly marketed as Avodart, dutasteride is a BPH medication. It works a little differently than finasteride because it inhibits all three isoenzymes or subtypes of the 5-alpha reductase (instead of just two, like finasteride does).[7] Dutasteride is commonly used for BPH. It is prescribed off-label for treating androgenic alopecia.

Like Proscar (the finasteride taken for BPH), taking Avodart is going to help with hair loss as a side effect, and may even have better outcomes because of the higher dosage.

In fact, studies out of Asia are indicating that dutasteride may be a little more beneficial than finasteride in helping with hair loss.[8] While finasteride and dutasteride are both approved by the FDA, only finasteride is approved in the United States for treating hair

---

7   I. H. Boersma et al., "The effectiveness of finasteride and dutasteride used for 3 years in women with androgenetic alopecia," *Indian Journal of Dermatology, Venereology and Leprology*, vol. 80, no. 6 (November-December 2014), accessed August 6, 2019 on PubMed.gov, https://www.ncbi.nlm.nih.gov/pubmed/25382509.

8   Z. Zhou, S. Song, Z. Gao, J. Wu, J. Ma, and Y. Cui. "The efficacy and safety of dutasteride compared with finasteride in treating men with androgenetic alopecia: a systematic review and meta-analysis," *Clinical Interventions in Aging*, vol. 14 (February 20, 2019): 399–406, accessed February 10, 2020 on *PubMed. gov*, https://www.ncbi.nlm.nih.gov/pubmed/30863034.

loss in men and in women who are not of childbearing age since it can cause fetal side effects and harm. It can also be used off-label in women who are posthysterectomy or postmenopausal, although doing so is still controversial. Dutasteride is approved in South Korea and Japan for hair loss, and is sometimes used off-label in the US.

Patients taking finasteride or dutasteride need to let their urologist or other doctor know since it may alter (prostate-specific antigen) PSA levels when screening for prostate cancer.

Spironolactone. Spironolactone is commonly used in acne treatment for women. It can also be an effective solution for hair loss in women because it slows down oil production in the skin by affecting hormone levels. It's not an option for men. I'll talk more about spironolactone in chapter 6.

Oral Medication Side Effects

While most patients tolerate oral medications very well, there is a very small percentage of patients that find them intolerable. Everyone is different, but some of the side effects that you may experience include:

- **Initial shedding.** Within the first six months of taking these medications, it's not uncommon to see some increased shedding. It's believed that this happens because the hairs are encouraged to cycle more. The miniaturized hairs that are being replaced slow down and stop growing before being replaced by new, thicker hairs. That process appears as regress.

- **Sexual dysfunction.** The most feared side effect of these medications is sexual dysfunction, which includes decreased libido and erectile dysfunction. Around 2 to 4 percent of patients taking these medications experience problems. However, studies of these drugs when initially released found that 2 percent of study participants taking a placebo also had sexual dysfunction. That means that only 2 percent of people taking the medication actually had a sexual side effect.[9]

- **Other side effects.** A very small percentage of patients (less than 1 percent) have other side effects that include gynecomastia (0.4 percent), rashes or hives, mood changes, testicular pain, or fertility issues.

A note of caution by the FDA: In addition to affecting screening for prostate cancer, finasteride and dutasteride may potentially increase the risk of high-grade prostate cancer. And, as I mentioned, it's also not to be handled by females who are pregnant or may become pregnant due to risk of side effects to a fetus. Still, Propecia (finasteride) and the topical Rogaine are both FDA approved for hair loss. Dutasteride, meanwhile, is FDA approved for BPH, but used off-label for hair loss.

Do not donate blood for at least six months after taking these meds, especially dutasteride, since it has a longer half-life and there's a risk of the blood being used by a female patient.

In my practice, we have patients review these side effects and potential side effects, and we invite questions and provide answers before we begin treatment.

Our review includes discussion of the rare post-finasteride syndrome. Side effects of this syndrome reportedly include more

---

9   G. A. Zakhem, J. E. Goldberg, C. C. Motosko, B. E. Cohen, R. S. Ho. "Sexual dysfunction in men taking systemic dermatologic medication: A systematic review," *Journal of the American Academy of Dermatology*, vol. 81, no. 1(July 2019): 163–172, accessed February 10, 2020 on *PubMed.gov*, https://www.ncbi.nlm. nih.gov/pubmed/30905792.

long-term loss of libido, changes in genital sensitivity, and erectile dysfunction. But to some degree, this syndrome is controversial because often other factors leading to hair loss are also occurring, such as aging, hormonal changes, and stress. So the medication may not be the sole cause of the problems, or even be a part of the problem at all.

In spite of the side effects and some controversy, oral medications have proven to be very effective in the patients we treat.

Natural Medications

Some people prefer to try natural DHT blockers and other medications for hair loss.

Some that may be helpful include the following:

- Saw palmetto is made from palm tree berries. It is a natural enzyme blocker that lowers DHT levels. It is also used for BPH treatment, but it is not to be taken with any prescription DHT blocker such as finasteride.

- Chinese herbs, including He Shoue Wu and Dabao.

- Horsetail extract.

- Nutrafol, a drug-free, natural hair loss supplement.

Other products advertised to help with hair loss that may or may not help include the following:

- Aloe vera.

- DHEA. This may even cause hair loss.

- Fava beans.

- Olive oil.

- Wheatgrass.

LOW LASER LIGHT THERAPY (LLLT)

Low laser light therapy (LLLT), also known as a laser cap, is another type of nonsurgical treatment.

Lasers are a specialized kind of light that target what are known as chromophores in tissue. Chromophores include melanin, which is the pigment in the skin and hair follicles; hemoglobin in blood; and water that is naturally within the tissue.

LLLT was developed in Hungary in the 1960s and initially used to stimulate a healing response in wounds. It was found to decrease inflammation and help with chronic pain.

Initially, laser devices for hair loss were combs, brushes, or bands. Today, we use laser caps, which are like baseball caps. In my practice, we partner with the Capillus brand of laser caps. You wear the Capillus cap at home for six minutes a day. There are also other caps that are worn less frequently but for longer periods of time and may require office visits. The lasers are absorbed superficially in the skin to target hair follicles, which are only five or six millimeters into the scalp. Although the biomechanism and the positive effects are not completely understood, there are some different theories about how laser therapy works.

In general, it's thought that the lasers shift the hairs more into the growing phase so they're staying in the growing phase longer and then resting for a shorter period of time. If you're getting those miniaturized hairs to grow thicker and fuller for a longer time, it gives the appearance of much more hair and coverage. At the cellular level, other metabolic changes may be helping the follicles absorb nutrients better. That may happen through increased circulation and oxygenation. Again, enhancing blood flow and circulation to hair follicles keeps them happy, healthy, and living longer while improving hair quality, stimulating regrowth, and increasing hair shaft diameter.[10] However, like other nonsurgical treatments, LLLT is not designed to grow new hair follicles. LLLT works best on androgenic alopecia, but it is also a viable treatment for women.

In addition to the take-home cap, there are also in-office lasers that are a little stronger. Some theoretical advantages are that they may be more precise or a little less stressful than the do-it-yourself, at-home treatment. If you're coming into the office to get the laser done, it can be monitored more regularly by the physician. But we've seen success with patients that do the treatment at home who were committed to a daily routine. With do-it-yourselfers, we monitor the progress every few months to make sure that it's working.

To determine whether a laser cap may be effective, during the consult, we look closely at the scalp using magnifying glasses or a device known as a densitometer. If we see miniaturized hairs, and depending on whether there is a differential diagnosis and other factors, then we may talk about whether you're a good candidate for the treatment.

LLLT is also very helpful in post-op healing after we transplant grafts. We find it to be very effective at helping the wound healing process and even helping grafts grow a little bit faster and fuller.

I can't say enough on how well I was treated Dr. Angelos was very professional and knowledgeable on all my concerns and my expectation. This is my second hair restoration procedure. The first one I had done was

---

10　Pinar Avci, et al., "Low-level laser (light) therapy (LLLT) in skin: stimulating, healing, restoring," *Seminars in Cutaneous Medicine and Surgery*, vol. 32, no. 1 (March 2013): 41–52, accessed August 6, 2019 on *PMC*, https://www.ncbi.nlm. nih.gov/pmc/articles/PMC4126803/.

with another doctor .. I was not impressed with the results so there was some hesitation on having another procedure done. After consulting with Dr. Angelos, I decided to have another hair restoration procedure. The experience and results were amazing. I can't thank Dr. Angelos enough for first class treatment I received from him and staff. I do plan on possibly having another procedure done in the future I will certainly have Dr. Angelos perform it as well. **—J. P.**

PLATELET-RICH PLASMA (PRP) TREATMENTS

Another nonsurgical medical treatment that has produced some positive results is platelet-rich plasma (PRP).

PRP is a concentrated source of the platelets and plasma from your own blood. During PRP, your whole blood is spun down to concentrate the platelets and to activate the release of their growth factors. These growth factors stimulate stem cells to help with wound healing. Think of a simple cut: as your blood clots, the platelets release growth factors to signal all the other tissue to come in and help heal the wound. By extracting those growth factors from your blood, they can be applied specifically to your wounds to enhance healing. The use of PRP scalp injections with the growth factors can also stimulate hair follicles, triggering growth and promoting neovascularization (the formation of new blood vessels) and improved hair growth characteristics.[11]

---

11   C. O. Uebel, J. B. da Silva, D. Cantarelli, and P. Martins, "The role of platelet plasma growth factors in male pattern baldness surgery," *Plastic and Reconstructive Surgery*, vol. 118, no. 6 (November 2006): 1458–66, accessed August 6, 2019, on *PubMed.gov*, https://www.ncbi.nlm.nih.gov/pubmed/17051119.

There are more than twenty different growth factors in platelets, and delving into them is a little scientific, but some of them include:

- PDGF, platelet-derived growth factor

- TGF, transforming growth factor

- VEGF, vascular endothelial growth factor

- IGF, insulin-like growth factors

- EGF, epidermal growth factor

PRP is not a new treatment. It was developed in the seventies and eighties and was initially popularized in oral and orthopedic surgery to help with wound healing. For oral surgery, it was used during dental implant procedures. In orthopedics, it helped to heal the union of bone fractures.

As a medical student, I conducted research with PRP in orthopedic surgery, and I wrote a review article on PRP for the medical university's orthopedic journal. Although I didn't ultimately go into orthopedic surgery, I find it interesting to see PRP in my current field of facial plastic surgery and hair restoration. It's been popularized for aesthetic-type treatments to improve skin tone and quality, especially of the face. These treatments include dermaplaning, microneedling, and what's known as a "vampire facelift," which involves injecting PRP into the face to fill out wrinkles.

Today, PRP is also being used for treating various types of alopecia, especially androgenic alopecia. It has been shown to be effective, although it remains controversial and does not work in all patients, so careful patient selection is important. Some of the studies of PRP for alopecia have shown:

- Growth factors from PRP had a significant effect on hair bulbs or follicles without side effects during treatment period and for twelve months after.[12]

- Several studies have found that PRP is safe, cost-effective, and nonallergic and that it can be used as an adjunct in the treatment of androgenic alopecia.[13]

- PRP can improve growth of transplanted follicles.[14]

It may be helpful to think of PRP as like a fertilizer for the hair follicles, including newly transplanted hair follicles or even those hair follicles that are miniaturized. Think about a plant that's not getting enough nutrients and sun to stimulate growth. In the same way, if we stimulate some of those wimpy, dying hair follicles using PRP along with LLLT, we can wake them up and get them growing more, growing healthier, and keep them growing longer.

We use PRP routinely at the time of transplant surgery because of its general effect, but also because of its effect on helping improve the growth of the newly grafted hairs.

PRP treatment starts by drawing whole blood, typically from the arm. Then it's processed or spun down in a centrifuge to activate the platelets and extract the PRP. The whole blood is drawn into a vacuum tube that contains reagents that separate the platelet-rich

---

12 Pietro Gentile et al., "The Effect of Platelet-Rich Plasma in Hair Regrowth: A Randomized Placebo-Controlled Trial," *Stem Cells Translational* Medicine, vol. 4, no. 11 (November 2015): 1317–1323, accessed August 6, 2019 on *PMC*, https://www.ncbi.nlm.nih.gov/pmc/articles/PMC4622412/#B4.

13 Nitin D. Chaudhari, Yugal K. Sharma, Kedar Dash, and Palak Deshmukh, "Role of Platelet-rich Plasma in the Management of Androgenetic Alopecia," *International Journal of Trichology*, vol. 4, no. 4 (October–December 2012): 291–292, accessed August 6, 2019 on *PMC*, https://www.ncbi.nlm.nih.gov/pmc/articles/PMC3681120/.

14 Suruchi Garg, "Outcome of Intra-operative Injected Platelet-rich Plasma Therapy During Follicular Unit Extraction Hair Transplant: A Prospective Randomised Study in Forty Patients," *Journal of Cutaneous and Aesthetic Surgery*, vol. 9, no. 3 (July–September 2016): 157–164, accessed August 6, 2019, on *PMC*, https://www.ncbi.nlm.nih.gov/pmc/articles/PMC5064679/.

plasma from the rest of the blood and then activate the release of their growth factors. The platelet-rich plasma is then injected into the scalp. The injections can be done with or without numbing the scalp. It's a little like Botox injections. Some patients tolerate them just fine, but others prefer to be numbed first. I let patients decide whichever they would prefer.

As part of hair restoration using PRP, we ask patients not to take certain anti-inflammatory medication, especially a few days after the treatment because we want it to create some degree of inflammatory response locally in the scalp for it to be most effective.

We generally recommend doing a series of PRP injections. For example, we do days zero, thirty, sixty, and ninety, or basically every month for three or four months. Then we do the injections every six months to try to maintain the growth. The reason for the series of injections is that we're trying to capture the hairs in their growing cycle. Not all the hairs are simultaneously growing, transitioning, resting; they are all in different phases of that cycle. If we treat the whole scalp with PRP treatment today, we're capturing those hairs in their growing cycle, but we're missing the ones that are transitioning or resting. By doing a series, we're capturing all phases of the cycle.

Since it's using your own blood and blood products, PRP is a very safe treatment. There's no chance for allergic reaction from the blood. However, some of the potential side effects with PRP are the same as with any injection. Those include bruising at the site where the blood is drawn, pain at the site of the injection, or bleeding or injury to a blood vessel or nerve that causes a temporary sensitivity or numbness. Far less likely is the side effect of permanent numbness.

THE MORE, THE BETTER

In general, the more you can do, the better when it comes to medical treatments. Those that I've mentioned in this chapter work in synergy. So, if you can do a combination of a topical or an oral along with a laser and PRP, you're probably going to get better results than just trying one treatment. For the best results, you must also commit to the treatment for life.

With any of the medical treatments or procedures that I've discussed in this chapter, the key is to be patient. It can take months to begin to see results, and it's best to give those results a year to really determine whether the treatment is working.

Whatever the treatment, we monitor patients over time to gauge results. The frequency of those visits really depends on the treatment, the patient, and the results we're seeing.

But everyone has an idea of how much time they want to spend on hair treatment, what side effects they're willing to tolerate, and how much they're will to spend out of their budget. Again, medications and nonsurgical treatments generally don't produce new hair follicles in thinning or balding areas. Where the follicles have stopped growing, topicals, orals, laser therapy, or PRP are just not going to be all that effective. At that point, your main options are surgical or transplantation.

CHAPTER 4

SURGICAL OPTIONS

*E*ven with all the options we have available today for creating far more natural-looking results, people often equate hair restoration to the hair plugs that produced "doll's hair" in the past. But some of the surgical hair transplant procedures we have today can fill in sparse areas and make the hair look more natural, nearly eliminating plugs as a treatment option today.

When hair loss is very advanced, medical treatments may restore some hair, but the only way to get significant and noticeable results—permanent results—is with a surgical option. Although patients with hair loss at Norwood II or III can be candidates for less extensive surgical procedures, for patients with advanced male pattern baldness—no real hair on top or basically a IV, V, or VI on the Norwood Scale—the best option is transplantation. When surgery is an option, we take into account progressive hair loss.

Surgical options are based on the principle of donor dominance, the concept that hair harvested from the back and sides of the scalp can be transplanted to the top and it will grow and remain there permanently. Even if all you have left is a little horseshoe ring around the sides and back of your head, that hair can be transplanted to the front and top, and it can live there permanently.

FACTORS TO CONSIDER

Determining whether a patient is a candidate for a procedural treatment versus a medical or surgical treatment comes down to several factors.

Androgenic alopecia (AGA) or male pattern baldness. This is really the main diagnosis to treat with transplantation surgery. Although other medical conditions like those I've mentioned in earlier chapters can make someone a candidate for transplantation, too, the vast majority of men seeking treatment are experiencing androgenic alopecia.

Enough donor hair. In order to be a candidate for hair transplantation, there must be enough donor hair, and there must be good density in the donor area. Sometimes, there is limited donor hair because of too many previous transplants or too much scarring in the donor area from trauma or for other reasons. Without enough donor hair, you won't get sufficient coverage—a limited transplant (using a limited amount of donor hair) means limited results. Trying to do a limited transplant can almost be worse than doing nothing at all because it can look really unnatural. Similar to other types of transplants, such as organs, transplanting from another source (such as someone else's hair) would mean a lifetime of taking immunosuppressive drugs and high risk for infection. So, unfortunately, using a different donor is not an option in hair transplantation.

Normal scalp mobility and flexibility. The scalp should be loose and flexible as opposed to tight or scarred, especially if considering FUT/strip surgery. Some people have tightness in the scalp due to muscle tension from temporomandibular joint dysfunction (TMJ) or other causes. Scarring from trauma or a scalp condition can also cause tightness, where the scalp simply isn't flexible and has some degree of immobility. Genetics and ethnicity may also contribute to scalp mobility; some patients just tend to have a softer, mushier scalp that moves around the bone better than others. Aging also contributes to laxity of the scalp, as does sun exposure—multiple sunburns can make the scalp tighter.

Hair thickness. The thickness or caliber of the hair shaft itself can determine whether someone is a better candidate for transplant. Medium to coarse hair is better than thin or fine hair for transplantation. A graft of fine or thin hair just doesn't look nearly as good as a transplant of medium to coarse hair. However, every patient is evaluated on a case-by-case basis to determine the best treatment. With fine hair, for instance, we need to do more grafts and pack them in tighter, so we have to adjust expectations about the result—a person with thinner hair shafts may not end up with the same thicker, fuller-looking head of hair as someone with thicker hair shafts.

Realistic expectations. This may be the most important point in determining candidate eligibility. There must be a good relationship and understanding between the patient and the doctor, especially in regard to the patient's goals and expectations. It comes down to big-picture planning—what's the ultimate goal to address the progression of hair loss? For younger patients, that may mean trying medical treatments plus minor surgery. For older patients with more advanced loss, we'll look at surgery to try to treat hair loss, use medical treatment to prevent further loss, and then also potentially plan for a subsequent procedure down the road to address more hair loss or ideal density as long as they have enough donor supply.

THE TRUTH ABOUT HAIR RESTORATION

MYTH: All types of hair transplantation look unnatural.

TRUTH: Today's hair restoration options include transplant treatments that look and perform like natural hair.

Unfortunately, there are some people who are *not* good candidates for surgical hair transplant. These include:

- Men who have diffuse unpatterned alopecia (DUPA). This is not the typical male pattern baldness and results in low donor supply.

- Patients with low donor supply of hair.

- Patients with severe scarring in the scalp.

- Patients with scalp tightness.

- Patients with a history of vascular injuries to the scalp.

- Patients with a history of radiation exposure for cancer treatment or other reasons. Radiation causes hair loss, fibrosis, and scarring, and it depletes blood supply.

- Women that have diffused thinning all over.

Still, transplant solutions are the most advanced treatments we've seen to date—and they're vastly improved from where we started with treatments for thin or balding hair.

HAIR TRANSPLANTS—WE'VE COME A LONG WAY

Surgical treatments for hair loss date back as far as two hundred years—the first hair transplant was described in 1822 in Germany by a medical student, Johann Dieffenbach. His initial studies involved using hair, feathers, and skin to perform transplants on animals.

Later in the 1800s, treatment started involving **scalp flaps**, which were primarily done to reduce scarring-type alopecia. The scalp flap procedure was pioneered by Herman Tillman, MD, as a way of reducing the alopecia in a round patch on the scalp due to trauma, injury, medical treatment, or other reasons. The procedure involves making pinwheel incisions around the alopecia, peeling back the pinwheels, and then suturing them back together. The procedure reduces the size of the bald area by bringing the hair-bearing skin and scalp closer together.

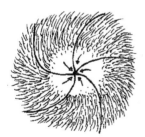

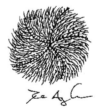

In the 1930s, there were advancements in hair transplantation by Japanese doctors, but this work was not read by the Western world because it was published in a rare dialect that was not widely understood. Among these advances were very natural-looking single hair grafts by Dr. Tamara, starting in 1937, which were essentially the precursor to modern follicular unit extraction (FUE) hair transplant techniques that we use today. (I'll explain FUE in more detail later in the chapter.) In 1939, Dr. Okuda used small graft transplants (one to five millimeters) for scarring and congenital alopecia. Dr. Okuda even published a landmark series of articles, "Clinical and Experimental Study of Living Hair Transplantation," in the *Japanese Journal of Dermatology*, which unfortunately wasn't widely distributed or read. Drs. Tamara and Okuda, who used their techniques on burn victims during wartime, are largely credited with some of the early research and understanding of hair transplantation.

Unfortunately, because of the language barrier and the collapse of Japan following the war, their techniques were not taken up by doctors in the United States at that time. If we had understood the research back then, hair transplantation would likely have taken an entirely different path.

Instead, it wasn't until the 1950s and '60s that Dr. Norman Orentreich popularized punch grafting and plug techniques, which used four-millimeter round punches to harvest grafts containing fifteen to twenty-four hairs from the occipital scalp (the very back of the scalp) and transplanted them in rows to the front and midscalp areas. These large grafts left the donor area riddled with "shotgun" scars and the recipient areas only partially treated. As hair loss progressed, patients were often left with exposed, unnatural-looking grafts.

Dr. Orentreich's techniques employed the principle that he introduced in 1959 in his paper, "Autografts in Alopecia and Other

Selected Dermatological Conditions," published in the *Annals of the New York Academy of Science*. Again, donor dominance is the principle that hair taken from the donor site in the sides and back of the scalp will grow permanently if transplanted to balding areas on the top and front of the scalp. That's because the donor hairs are taken from areas of the scalp that are resistant to the effects of DHT (the sides and back), even though the area that they are transplanted in (front and top) are susceptible to DHT.

In his paper, Dr. Orentreich also explained the principle of recipient dominance—hairs will take on slight and subtle characteristics of the area where they are implanted. In other words, hairs taken from the sides and back of the scalp and moved to the front may slowly, over time, start to take on the characteristics of the hairs in that front area. For example, if someone generally has wavier hair in the front than they do on the back and the sides of their scalp, the straighter donor hair implanted in the front may become a wavy over time to match the other hair in the area.

Similarly, hair transplanted from the scalp to the eyebrows will change characteristics over time. Generally, scalp hair grows a lot faster and thicker than eyebrow hair. But once implanted, factors in the soft tissue and cells signal the hairs to grow slower and finer, just like eyebrow hair.

It's the same with body hair moved to the scalp. Although transplanting body hair to the scalp is not as common, occasionally, coarser, wavy chest hair may be transplanted to the scalp. Over time, the hair will grow a little bit more like scalp hair than chest hair.

In addition to transplants that took advantage of the concept donor dominance, other treatments continued to be developed over the years.

In 1969, Dr. Jose Juri of Argentina introduced the first large pedicle flap. Also known as a Juri flap, this procedure lifts hair-bearing scalp from side and back of the head, and then drapes it over the front of the scalp. This is not a procedure commonly used in the United States these days, but it is still performed by a few surgeons internationally.

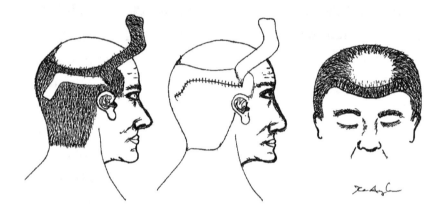

Some of the problems with the Juri flap procedure include the following:

- **High failure rate** due to lack of blood supply to the flap. The flap of skin that's moved is connected to an artery, a vein, and some other vasculature. It can be tricky to keep the blood supply to that flap intact when moving it. If the blood supply is compromised, the whole flap could die, and you'll lose all that hair-bearing skin.

- **Scarring** in the donor area and in front where the flap is moved. This can be especially problematic for patients who are prone to what's called hypertrophic or keloid scarring (red and raised scarring) because it can look very unnatural.

- **Unnatural appearance in the front** because the density and direction of the hair growth is not typical for what you would normally see in that area. Since it is the hair brought from the side and back of the scalp, it appears to transition abruptly, going from denser hair in the front of the scalp to thinner, balding hair just behind that front area.

- **High risk for complications**, especially bleeding, nerve injury, and numbness beyond the desired aesthetic outcome, since it is such an invasive procedure.

In the 1970s, **scalp reduction surgery** became more popular because of Drs. Guy and Bernard Blanchard and Dr. L. Lee Bosley (whose name you have likely heard). These doctors performed what was termed male pattern reduction for more advanced thinning and hair loss, around IV or V on the Norwood scale.

Like scalp flaps, scalp reduction surgery requires good scalp mobility. The way scalp reduction works is by excising a Y-shaped area out of the crown to remove as much bald skin as possible without causing too much scarring, and bringing together more hair-bearing scalp to provide more coverage.

Scalp reduction has largely fallen out of favor as a surgical option except for patients who are not candidates for any other options or as an adjunct to some other types of hair transplantation techniques. That's because problems with scalp reduction include scarring where the skin has been stretched, long-term numbness, risk of complications, and long recovery time.

In 1975, Dr. O'Tar Norwood, a dermatologist and hair transplant surgeon, created the Norwood Scale, which is still in use today. His scale is based on a study of one thousand male hairlines, but it is actually a revision of a classification developed nearly a quarter century earlier by an anatomist, Hamilton, who studied hair patterns in three hundred men. The late 1970s and into the 1980s was a transition period in hair restoration, as tools used by surgeons began to allow for progressively smaller grafts. Minigrafts during this time involved four to twelve hairs. Micrografts involved one to four hairs. Minigrafts and micrografts were not necessarily harvested by what are known as follicular units (FUs), which are naturally growing groups of one, two, three, or four hairs within the scalp.

SURGERY USING FOLLICULAR UNITS

Over time, a couple of other types of surgery were developed, and these are still used today: follicular unit transfer (FUT) and follicular unit extraction (FUE).

Both involve follicular units, or FUs, a term that was first defined in the early 1980s by Dr. John Headington in his paper, "Transverse Microscopic Anatomy of the Human Scalp." Transplantation involved dividing up hairs along the cleavage planes of one to four hairs.

Back then, gaining a close look at the hair during transplantation was done with a jeweler's loupe. Since those provided a very limited amount of magnification, follicular units were often transected, or damaged, during harvest. Transecting is when a hair is severed above the follicle or bulb, rendering it useless for transplant. The procedure was called mini-micro grafting, and the high transection rate made it impossible to achieve the density that hair transplant patients can achieve today.

Follicular unit transfer (FUT). In the 1990s, FU grafting from what was known as "strip harvesting" became the new standard in transplantation. With the introduction of the stereoscopic dissecting microscope, Dr. Bobby Limmer discovered that a strip of scalp and hair taken from the back of the scalp could be divided up into those naturally occurring FUs. That allowed for more hairs to be harvested from the strip, resulting in more hairs to transplant than the traditional minigrafts or micrografts.

Known as follicular unit transfer (FUT), or more commonly "strip surgery," this type of transplantation involves harvesting a strip of follicles from the back of the scalp to use for filling in areas on the front and sides. The strip includes skin and all the hair follicles within it. The strip is then cut into small pieces, sort of a like a loaf of bread that is sliced and then each slice cut into smaller squares.

Once the strip is removed from the scalp, then the scalp above and below the strip must be stretched and sutured together. That can lead to some problems, especially if the suture is not closed meticulously or well.

The surgery leaves a scar approximately a centimeter or two in vertical height along the back of the scalp, nearly from ear to ear. This treatment is not used as often today because most patients don't want the linear scar along the back of the scalp.

This is where plastic surgeons are at a distinct advantage, in my opinion. Even over dermatologists and other hair transplant surgeons as far as being meticulous about closure—and during the surgery itself. In addition to regularly performing surgery on the scalp for various reasons, I've published a paper on forehead and scalp reconstruction for skin cancer defects. I'm biased, but I do think that all my experience with scalp surgery gives me an artistic edge

> All my experience with scalp surgery gives me an artistic edge over other hair restoration professionals who don't perform surgery.

over other hair restoration professionals who don't perform surgery. As a plastic surgeon, I specialize in reconstructive surgery for all areas above the shoulders.

There are some advantages and disadvantages to FUT. First the advantages:

- It's generally less expensive than follicular unit extraction (FUE), which I will explain next. The lower costs are mainly because it's the less time consuming and doesn't necessarily involve some of the technologies that I will explain later in the book.

- With FUT, we can do more grafts per session, often three to four thousand. That makes it potentially a better option for someone with advanced hair loss.
Now, the disadvantages:

- The long, linear scar, which can be visible with short hair. A lot of patients complain that, once they've had strip surgery, they can't wear their hair as short as they like to because the scar will be visible.

- Sensitivity, numbness, or pain at the scar. This can be temporary or, for some patients, chronic.

- Longer recovery time than the more minimally invasive FUE techniques.

- Activity restrictions during recovery time. It can take up to two weeks to recover, and during that time, we ask patients to limit exercise or exertional activity for risk of opening the wound or having a hematoma or major bleeding.

- Higher risk of complications. Since it's a little more invasive than FUE, bleeding can be a complication.

FUT ultimately evolved into a procedure used more commonly today known as follicular unit extraction (FUE).

FUE vs FUT

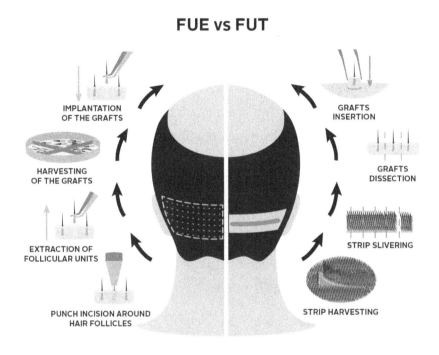

Follicular unit extraction (FUE). This type of transplant was first described by Masumi Inaba in Japan in 1988, and it was the first time a very small, one-millimeter punch began being used to extract FUs. Manual punches come in a variety of sizes today, all measuring at or under one millimeter in size. They're still very useful for performing biopsies of the scalp and of hair follicles. Some surgeons still prefer using them for hair transplantation because they feel like the tactile feedback helps them get really good results. Manual punches are also useful for small test sessions, such as testing a certain number of grafts to see how well a patient does with harvesting or how well those grafts might take in a previously scarred transplant area.

In 1989, a Dr. Ray Woods conducted FUE on patients in Australia, and seven years later, he was filmed performing the procedure for a program known as *Good Medicine*. In 2002, more than a decade after it was introduced, FUE was the topic of a ground-breaking medical article, "Follicular Unit Extraction: Minimally Invasive Surgery for Hair Transplantation," by William R. Rassman and Robert M. Bernstein. In the paper, they described exclusively using FUE for hair transplants.

With FUE, instead of making a big strip scar, we individu-ally extract follicular units. Once the individual follicular units are extracted, they're counted and sorted, and then implanted into the scalp, just like with FUT. Other than the harvesting, FUE is a very similar process to FUT (strip surgery).

Advantages of FUE include:

- It is minimally invasive since the follicles are harvested indi-vidually using small, one-millimeter punches.

- No linear scar.

- Minimal discomfort.

- Short recovery with fewer activity restrictions. With FUE, you can return to work and activities sooner, typically within a day or two.

- No sutures/staples to be removed.

- Results appear more natural because there is no scar in the donor area.

- Less potential for damage to surrounding follicular units.
  The disadvantages of manual FUE:

- Not everyone is a good candidate for FUE. One of the biggest reasons a person may not be a good candidate is because of curly donor hair. It's difficult to extract individual follicular units that are curlicued under the skin.

- More expensive, mainly because of the time involved.

- Time consuming—it can take more than one session to transplant all the individual follicles.

- Trimming the donor area. The donor area must be trimmed very short to be able to identify and extract those individual follicular units. That's a bit of a psychological challenge for some patients who are already concerned about their hair loss, and now we're asking them to trim their hair even shorter. Plus, they often want to be private about having the procedure, so they sometimes take time off work and more or less hide out until the hair starts to grow back.

- High rate of collateral damage. During the harvesting process, it's possible to damage adjacent follicle units. If two or three units are harvested, but only one unit survives the process to be transplanted, then those other units are destroyed permanently—they will never grow back. That can result in overharvesting of the donor site. This is where the surgeon's artistic ability is a real advantage—a more experienced provider is far less likely to overharvest from the donor area.

Originally, FUE was a manual process, but over time, it has become more automated and efficient due to advances in the punches. Some of the early innovations with automated punches were adaptations of dental drills and other motorized types of punches. These sped up the transplantation process and included a semiautomated punch known as a direct hair implanter, which performed the entire implant procedure all at once.

Later, John Cole patented a device limiting the depth of the punch insertion and described the follicular isolation technique. There was limited adoption of the device due to the high risk of transecting the follicle during harvesting because of the sharp punch. The punch also required the graft to be tethered below the sharp dissection, which made it more difficult to extract. Plus, the device never really became commercially available.[15]

In 2005, Dr. James Harris of Denver developed what he described in a paper as "The S.A.F.E. System for FUE." S.A.F.E., which stands for Surgically Advanced Follicular Extraction, was a major advance in FUE devices. It is a two-step system that uses a manual **sharp punch** to score the surface of the skin and then a rotating **dull punch** to dissect deeper into the tissue to avoid transection of follicles. This two-step system was to become the basis for the future mechanism of robotic FUE.[16] The goal of the S.A.F.E. system was to try to limit damage or transection of the hair follicles.

There are several advantages to the S.A.F.E. system. It can be more efficient and quicker than some of the manual extraction techniques, depending on the operator's experience. The dull punch slows down as it penetrates deeper into tissue to avoid damage to follicles. It can give good graft production rates and low transection rates; basically, that means it's very good at helping us harvest fewer hairs and getting higher yield with the hairs that we harvest. It helps minimize the number of other hairs that are damaged during the harvesting process.

---

15   Walter P. Unger et al., eds. *Hair Transplantation*, (London: Informa Healthcare, 2011).

16   J. A. Harris. "The S.A.F.E. System: New Instrumentation and Methodology to Improve Follicular Unit Extraction (FUE)," *Hair Transplant Forum International*, vol. 14, no. 5(2004):157, 163–4.

One of the potential downsides of the S.A.F.E. system is when the angles of the follicles are not ideal, because the dull punches can compress the skin and soft tissue. That can bury the grafts and make it harder or more traumatic to extract them, potentially damaging them.

But overall, the S.A.F.E. system is a very good, very popular device. A lot of hair transplant surgeons would say that of all the automated or handheld FUE devices, S.A.F.E. is certainly one of the better, if not the best.

Another device is the NeoGraft, which is the brand name of a motorized punch device that extracts with a rotating sharp punch and collects the follicles by suction into a trap. That process can remove some of the tissue around the base of graft, potentially exposing it to mechanical injury and drying out of the graft. One way that some surgeons combat the drying issue is by removing the filter in the suction line. Then the grafts are suctioned down the tubing and into a saline bath.

NeoGraft requires a fair amount of operator intervention to keep the process functioning smoothly. Anyone with some training can use it—a technician, a nurse, a surgeon. But that's actually one of the downsides to it. Since its use depends heavily on the operator's abilities, transplant success can come down to the experience of the person performing the procedure.

Hair transplantation is very work-intensive and really requires a fair amount of artistry to design a hairline and transplant plan that looks at areas of more or less density, the best areas for harvest, the orientation of recipient sites, and the angles of future hair growth.

THE TRUTH ABOUT HAIR RESTORATION

MYTH: Hair restoration is an aggressive treatment involving a lot of scarring.

TRUTH: Transplantation involving extraction and implantation of follicular units is minimally invasive. There is far less discomfort, quick healing, and minimal scarring. You can even wear your hair short afterward, if you so choose.

While the tools available today make it possible for people with little training to perform hair restoration, the best outcomes come from surgeons with clinical and aesthetic skills. More than just having the right tools, you need an experienced provider who understands some of the best options for your specific needs and desires.

OTHER SURGICAL OPTIONS (PROCEED WITH CAUTION)

In addition to FUT and FUE, there are some other surgical procedures being performed to try to increase scalp circulation and alleviate tightness in the scalp.

One of these is known as a galeotomy, which is done more outside the United States. The galea is a layer deeper within the soft tissue of the scalp. A galeotomy makes small incisions to release or relax the galea layer to try to get the scalp to loosen up as a way of increasing circulation. Galeotomies are controversial, with many doctors and surgeons calling the procedure hocus-pocus because blood circulation in the scalp is actually above the galea. I tend to agree with those that say the procedure misses its target.

Other procedures that I've already discussed have also fallen out of favor, such as the scalp reduction techniques and Juri flaps. Those are generally, in my opinion, not good options, just because they're more invasive. You can get, in my opinion, better, more natural results with the advancement of FUE, minimally invasive techniques.

Again, a caveat: If a patient is just not a good candidate for FUE, or they don't want to undergo FUT, one of the other surgical procedures may be a good option.

For example, some African American men tend to have more mobility in their scalp. If an African American gentleman has only a small amount of crown baldness, then he might be a good candidate for a scalp reduction technique, just to make that area of the crown much smaller. Then, if that's not enough, we may do a small amount of transplanting around that scalp reduction. But in general, we really just don't recommend some of those more invasive techniques unless there are special circumstances.

The key is to find a practice that has many options available and individualizes the treatment to your specific needs and wants.

Since the ARTAS is the most advanced technology we have today for hair restoration, I've devoted the next chapter to explaining more about this amazing tool. While it's primarily used for harvesting in my practice, it's also a tool for site-making and implantation.

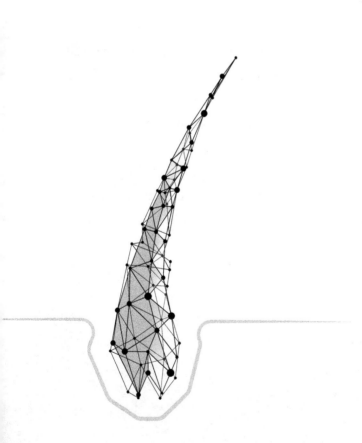

CHAPTER 5

ROBOTIC HAIR RESTORATION
WITH THE ARTAS iX

*P*atients often come to see me after having undergone a surgical hair transplant procedure and not being entirely happy with their results. One patient I helped even had two different strip scars—those lines at the back of the scalp where hair has been harvested and then implanted up front.

Usually, patients who have had strip surgery don't want the same procedure again because they want to avoid another scar. But they want more hair restored either because their hair loss has progressed or they don't have the density they want.

We also see patients who have never been treated, yet they know someone else with a scar, and they don't want that for themselves. They want to wear their hair short, and they don't want to have a hairless line showing across the back of their scalp. Or maybe they've actually done some research on FUE, found robotic treatment, and want to know more about it. Again, strip surgery and FUT transplants are falling out of favor. We still use them in some cases, but most people want FUE.

ARTAS DEVELOPMENT

When the ARTAS System was launched in 2011 for clinical use, it was designed as a tool only for harvesting. In 2012, more automated settings were added, which helped to improve the user experience. In 2013, the speed of harvesting was improved. Then, in 2015, the Artist Hair Studio, a digital, preoperative planning technology, was introduced to give the provider an extra tool for designing the patient's treatment. A second generation of the app came with the 2016 (8x) version of the ARTAS graft selection algorithm added. But one of the biggest advancements came in 2017 with the 9x version, which was an Advanced Vision System and one-touch that increased efficiency and improve site-making capabilities. The improvements to the 9x version made ARTAS really take off with providers. Now, with the iX version of the ARTAS, the unit has a more compact robotic arm and head and it is exceptional for harvesting, but it can also perform site-making and implantation.

EVOLUTION OF FUE TECHNOLOGIES

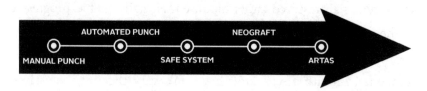

I am very happy and satisfied with my hair restoration experience with Dr. Angelos and the team at Charleston Plastic Surgery. Frankly, I was shocked that it went as smoothly as it did. Several of my friends have done hair restoration work with mixed experiences. For me, the robot ARTAS was the only way to go. The harvesting and planting of follicles went smoothly and healing was very fast. You could hardly tell the next day where they harvested the follicles. The staff is very professional and fun to work with making my hair restoration day a very positive experience. **—N. H.**

The ARTAS System offers the precision of robotics along with physician-assisted control. By that I mean the physician is able to control some of the parameters and depth of the needle, depth of the dull punch, and the angle of approach in harvesting. Ultimately, that leads to precision and accuracy of repeatable, good-follicle harvesting.

For the provider, treating with fully manual or semiautomated FUE, like with NeoGraft or the S.A.F.E. System, can present limitations because of eye strain, muscle fatigue, mental fatigue, and human error. As you can imagine, it can get very tedious and tiring to extract two thousand grafts, whether manually or with a handheld device. The 1,999th graft isn't going to be the quality as the first graft. That's the fundamental reason that robot technology came about—it was designed to create natural, reproducible results, especially in harvesting, while minimizing the damage to the surrounding follicles. The beauty of the ARTAS robotic system is that it really manages the repetitive work of extracting thousands of grafts in a single session, thereby minimizing physician fatigue and error, and lowering the potential to transect or damage the hair follicle.

Using robotics for critical aspects of FUE, such as harvesting and even site-making and implantation, has been a game changer for the industry, and the ARTAS Robotic Hair Transplant System is one of the most powerful tools we have for creating the most natural-looking outcomes.[17]

> The beauty of the ARTAS robotic system is that it really manages the repetitive work of extracting thousands of grafts in a single session, thereby minimizing physician fatigue and error, and lowering the potential to transect or damage the hair follicle.

One of the other big advancements with the iX is more selectivity with the grafts. It allows the provider to dial in the parameters of the robot and determine, for example, to skip single hairs or skip X number of single hairs. Single hairs work best in the front of the scalp, which is where they are naturally occurring. But farther back on the scalp, toward the crown, the single hairs transition to denser groups of two, three, and four hairs.

If we're doing a full hair transplant, let's say two thousand grafts, then we determine the number of singles we need for the front of the hairline, let's say two hundred, and then the remaining we'll harvest in groups of two, three, and four plus. If only the crown is being transplanted, then we want to get much more density. The robotic program allows us to skip single hairs and harvest FUs with more hairs. That's how to produce a much better result.

---

17   Robert M. Bernstein, and Michael B. Wolfeld, "Innovations in Robotic Hair Restoration," *Modern Aesthetics*, March/April 2018, accessed November 2, 2019, https://modernaesthetics.com/articles/2018-mar-apr-insert/innovations-in-robotic-hair-restoration.

UNPRECEDENTED RESULTS

The ARTAS iX computer software and its high-definition stereoscopic camera give physicians unprecedented accuracy, efficiency, and reproducibility in harvesting grafts for hair transplantation.

The system can analyze a hair in the scalp about sixty times per second. Compare that to a human doing manual FUE or handheld FUE: with our eyes and brain we can only process ten to twelve images per second.

The ARTAS iX also identifies and selects prime hair for harvesting. It detects and determines angles, thickness, and type of hair, resulting in high-quality grafts with fewer transections or damage to surrounding follicles.

The physician can also set what's known as site-spacing to very close parameters; for instance, in very high-density donor areas, we can get that site-spacing to as close as 1.6 millimeters. When it extracts an FU in an area, it flags that area with a circle and then will not harvest any additional hairs within that circle. We can set that site-spacing based on the density of the donor area.

The site-spacing feature is key to avoiding overharvesting, which tends to happen more with manual or handheld FUE. Overharvesting is when the operator has taken out too many grafts or, in the process of taking out the grafts has damaged the surrounding hair. Those extracted grafts or damaged follicles will not grow back—the damage is almost impossible to reverse, which is why our goal is to avoid overharvesting altogether.

It can also determine the correct depth of dissection and angle of approach during site-making and implantation. It can identify the location of existing hairs in the scalp, protect them, and make the recipient sites in between where hair needs to be added without damaging existing hairs.

BENEFITS OF ARTAS ROBOTIC HARVESTING

- **Uses a high-definition stereoscopic vision system** to analyze, monitor, and track each hair sixty times per second. Is far and away the best technology for harvesting.

- **ARTAS Artificial Intelligence** identifies and selects prime hair for harvesting. It detects and determines angles, thickness, and type of hair.

- **Physician-assisted robotic technology**, so the thousandth graft is the same quality as the first graft. Robots do not get fatigued.

- **Robotic precision** provides speed, accuracy, and reproducibility to create natural, permanent results.

- **Protects surrounding follicles** during harvest and site-making. It avoids damaging existing, healthy (permanent) hair.

- **Fast recovery** since robotics makes the process minimally invasive. Recovery is quick and easy, allowing you to get back to work and your daily activities quickly.

- **Minimal scarring**. There is no linear scar, and the very small scars created are typically not noticeable, even if you wear your hair very short.

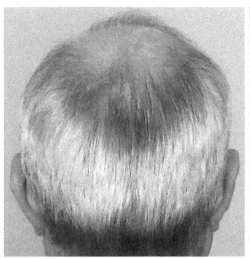
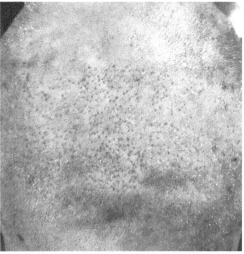
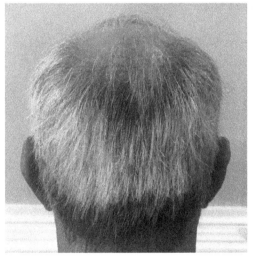

ARTAS harvesting (donor sites and healing)
before (top left), POD 1 R scalp,
POD 0 L scalp* after 6 months
*Harvesting is usually done all in one day, this case was done over
two days (note how quickly the right side is already healing)

As with any FUE procedure, hair must be cut to one millimeter
in length before the procedure. However, in many patients using a

robot for site-making, the natural, existing hairs are already growing back within a couple of weeks. Plus, with ARTIS iX, there is no linear scar left in the donor area. Any scarring in the donor area is not typically detectable, allowing you to wear your hair in any style you want.

But one of the features I love most about the robotic technology is that is allows me to spend more time with you, the patient, designing your hairline and understanding your goals and objectives.

THE ROBOTIC RESTORATION PROCEDURE

There's a common misconception that treatment with the ARTAS iX is a fully automated process—we just put you in a room with the robot and press "go." That's not the way it works. It's a physician-assisted system. Although it has AI, which determines dissection parameters (needle and core depth, and angle of approach), I personally operate the robot at the user interface to make the manual adjustments needed so that we're continually getting the best possible grafts for transplant.

For example, with each little harvest section of the scalp, we may extract ten or more grafts. Then I stop the robot and look at the grafts under a microscope to ensure that they're very high quality. If needed, I then adjust dissection parameters beyond the robot's AI. I keep doing that to dial in what we need the robot to do.

The harvest process itself involves a needle-and-punch mechanism where the needle scores the skin and the dull (to protect the hair follicles) rotating punch dissects deeper to harvest the follicles.

The robot doesn't completely extract the follicles out of the scalp during harvest. Instead, it very slightly lifts the follicles out of the scalp a few millimeters but leaves them in the skin. Then, we go back in and manually extract them. That's different than some of the handhelds, like NeoGraft, for example, which suctions the follicle all the way out into a trap, increasing the risk of overdrying the grafts. But with the ARTAS technology, the graft stays in the scalp longer, where it continues to get blood supply.

By leaving the grafts in the body for a longer period of time, we can avoid overprocessing them. Just like with any kind of transplant surgery—when an organ or skin graft is harvested, we don't want it to be without its blood supply for very long. How the grafts are handled depends on the provider: they are either extracted one small grid area at a time, or all the grafts needed for a transplant are extracted at once.

The robot is also ideal for "random" site-making when we're filling in around existing hair that needs to be protected. It can identify existing hairs on top of the scalp, and based on the design input to the robot, can evenly distribute the recipient sites.

THE TRUTH ABOUT HAIR RESTORATION

MYTH: It's often thought that "robotics" means we place a patient in the treatment room and let a machine do all the work.

TRUTH: The ARTAS robotics system is not a fully automated robot. We don't just put you in the room and press "go." It's physician-assisted. I personally run the robot at the user interface to make sure that we're getting the best possible grafts for transplant.

In my practice, we mainly use the robot for harvesting and some site-making. But I do a lot of manual site-making, especially where the scalp is highly curved, where the crown swirl pattern is unique, and where the angles are very sharp in the front of the scalp. In these areas, I prefer to use my artistic talent and expertise instead of relying entirely on the robot. While it's an amazing tool, it still has some limitations.

However, Venus Concept, which in 2019 purchased ARTAS maker Restoration Robotics, is always advancing this technology. Under the new ownership, the technology will continue to improve.

Even though there are many advantages to robotics, and people are often drawn to it, we want to be able to offer every type of treatment and do what's best for each patient. That includes treatment for women, for whom hair thinning and loss can be especially disheartening.

CHAPTER 6

HAIR RESTORATION FOR WOMEN

*W*hile hair thinning and loss is a distressing problem for many men, it's especially worrisome for women because it is less acceptable in society. Hair loss is especially devastating for younger women—it can make them feel less youthful, less attractive, less sexy. Yet up to 25 percent of women suffer hair thinning and loss.

But there is hope. In fact, we see quite a few women in my hair restoration clinic, and we offer a variety of treatments from medical to procedural to surgical.

Women who find themselves losing hair typically are very distraught when they come in to see us. Stereotypically, it's somewhat normal and even accepted for men to lose some of their hair. In men, hair loss typically happens along the lines of the Norwood classification scale that I've mentioned in earlier chapters—there are several defined patterns.

But in women, hair loss is initially less apparent; one of the first things that becomes noticeable is thinning in certain areas. Women largely discover they have a problem when they have trouble styling their hair. They find themselves trying to compensate for thinning by restyling. But over time, as the thinning progresses, they begin to realize that they actually have a problem—they're getting to the point that they can no longer cover up the loss. That's when they come to see us.

Women especially, it seems, don't like to view hair loss as a natural part of aging and something they can do nothing about. Yet many of our female patients tell us that is what they've been told by their primary care doctor: "You're just getting older. Hair loss is a natural part life. It's just something you have to deal with."

As with men, the challenge with women is to first figure out the culprit—what's causing the hair loss in the first place?

CAUSES OF HAIR LOSS IN WOMEN

With women, the potential causes of hair loss are vastly different than men. In nine out of ten men, androgenic alopecia is the cause of hair loss. But for women, there are a variety of reasons for hair loss, and they are not nearly as predictable.

Anemia, or low iron. Different kinds of anemia or low blood count can cause hair loss. These include iron deficiency anemia, which, as its name states, is caused by low iron levels in the blood. Women are more prone to low iron levels than men because of nutritional deficiencies, pregnancy, and other health issues.

Thyroid disease. Hypothyroid, or low thyroid, is more common in women than men. Having low thyroid levels can cause hair loss and thinning.

Weight loss. Crash diets that are especially extreme can cause hair loss. Primarily this includes any that are starvation based and lead to nutritional deficiencies. That can cause the body's stress response to kick in and lead to hair loss.

Autoimmune diseases. These are diseases where your immune system attacks your body. These are typically more common in women than in men, and some of them, because of their systemic nature, can cause hair loss. Autoimmune diseases include lupus, rheumatoid arthritis, Crohn's disease, Sjögren's syndrome, autoimmune thyroid, and others. Autoimmune diseases can also affect the gastrointestinal tract, leading to nutritional issues that can then cause hair loss.

Some medications. Some oral contraceptive pills can lead to hair loss because of their effect on a woman's hormones.

Postpartum alopecia. After pregnancy, the hormonal changes that a woman's body undergoes can ultimately lead to hair loss. That may be because estrogen levels really build up during pregnancy, which can actually help hair. So, while a woman is pregnant, she may notice more fullness in her hair because her hormones are pushing her hairs into the anagen or growth phase. After the pregnancy, her estrogen levels decline, which shifts her hair cycle from the anagen or growing phase to the resting or telogen phase. It's not a true telogen effluvium, where the all the hairs go into the resting phase, but many of them do.

Again, telogen effluvium Is when the hairs are not really growing; they appear to be dormant. That phase can last two to six months; on average, it lasts three or four months. During that time, it looks like there is some hair loss, but the follicles aren't really gone. They are resting under the skin. They start to grow back in three or four months. But they are very short, just a few millimeters long. It actually takes months to get to the normal length of a woman's hair. In fact, full recovery may take upward of a year—it can take that long before the hair looks normal again. And if the woman is nursing and breastfeeding, it can take even longer because it can take a while for the hormones to stabilize.

We see quite a few patients who are postpartum and wondering what's happening with their hair. We just reassure them that it's going to take time for their hair to return to normal, and usually we don't need to start treatments. Instead, we take a wait-and-see approach.

Menopause. Menopause-related hair loss is a much bigger deal for many women. This type of hair loss can affect more than 50 percent of women. Menopause-based hair loss happens because of the significant drop in estrogen that happens as a woman ages. That can put the hairs in a prolonged resting phase.

Usually patients having other issues with estrogen loss may benefit from supplementation, which may then also help with hair loss.

Now let's look at some of the patterns of female hair loss, including postmenopausal hair loss.

FEMALE PATTERN HAIR LOSS

As part of diagnosing a woman's specific condition before we begin any treatment, we perform a series of tests on female patients.

Since some of the causes of hair loss in women are medically based, as part of the initial consultation, we do a blood test known as a female alopecia panel. With that test, we're checking blood, thyroid, iron, and hormone levels, and we're screening for autoimmune diseases. We also perform a scalp biopsy to look for autoimmune conditions that can affect the scalp. Alopecia areata is a mimicker of female or male pattern hair loss that we want to evaluate and rule out. We also look for those scarring versus nonscarring conditions that I mentioned in chapter two. And we want to differentiate a true alopecia from telogen effluvium, which is that stress response that leads to temporary hair loss.

As with men, there are some specific patterns of hair loss in women. When a woman has thinning or hair loss, it's not simply androgenic alopecia, like it is most of the time with men.

Here are some of the patterns of hair loss in women.

Classic pattern. The classic female pattern loss is different than in men. In women, the classic pattern tends to spare the anterior hairline, or the front centimeter or two of the hairline. Behind that is where thinning and loss usually occurs in women. Typically, women do not lose a lot of hair at the crown. The classic pattern occurs in around 10 percent of women.

Diffuse alopecia (hair loss). This is a more devastating type of hair loss in women. It involves thinning all over the scalp, including the sides and back (the areas of donor hair). Diffuse hair loss is more common in postmenopausal women, but it can happen in younger women as well. Women experiencing this type of loss often say that they're afraid they're going to lose all their hair: "Doctor, what am I going to do? I feel like I'm really going to go bald," we often hear. These women may already be wearing hairpieces or wigs to cover up their loss.

Perimenopause. Perimenopausal hair loss can start in a woman's thirties or forties. This pattern is usually like the classic pattern, worse in the front just behind the hairline. But it progresses a little more and can include the crown. Perimenopausal hair loss can develop very slowly, unlike hair loss in men, which typically progresses at a steady rate. This pattern tends to be relatively stable by the time it's diagnosed and it stays relatively stable until menopause, and then it accelerates to more of the diffuse hair loss pattern.

Diffuse unpatterned alopecia. This is very similar to diffuse hair loss in general. *Female genetic alopecia* and *senile alopecia* are two types of diffuse unpatterned alopecia. These are typically caused by genetics and aging, respectively.

Female pattern loss. This may be caused by a genetic predisposition and is significantly different from male pattern loss. It is not just androgenic alopecia. This pattern is postmenopausal and involves diffuse thinning just behind the normal hairline and extending beyond the crown and all the way to the back of the head. These patients often have significant levels of miniaturization on the back and sides of the scalp, so unfortunately, they are not good candidates for transplantation because they do not have good density or quality hair in the harvest area.

Some women may have an excess of male sex hormones, which is what causes androgenic alopecia. But most of the time, when we do laboratory tests, we find that a woman's hormone levels are normal. However, as mentioned earlier, the loss of the protective effect of estrogen over time may be a factor that leads to thinning. Some women with female pattern loss do well with estrogen supplementation.

In my opinion, it is a combination of genetic predisposition and hormonal factors around menopause that leads to the patterns of diffuse and genetic alopecia.

Male pattern baldness. Although it is less common, male pattern baldness occurs in about 15 percent of women. When this occurs, it is typically a result of aging, not because of hormone loss from menopause or pregnancy. This hair loss looks very much like the hair loss in men and includes temporal recession, just like seen in guys. With male pattern baldness, women typically don't get as much loss in the crown, but they can. But the good news is these patients are really good candidates for transplantation. They have a good, stable, high-density donor area, and they just need to add density and volume to areas of temporal recession or some early thinning through the top or the crown. I'll talk more about this later in the chapter.

When a woman has male pattern baldness, then it is better to classify her loss using the Norwood Scale. But outside of that condition, there are other classification scales to use in diagnosing women.

THE LUDWIG AND OTHER CLASSIFICATION SCALES

The classification scale often used for women is known as the Ludwig Classification Scale.[18] The Ludwig scale was identified based on a study of 468 women, and it includes three types:

- **Type I.** This is a mild widening of the width of the part and some early diffuse thinning. This type occurs in 80 percent of women with hair loss.

- **Type II.** This is a moderate widening of the width of the part and diffuse thinning over the top of the scalp. This type occurs in 15 percent of women.

18 Gomez, *Hair Loss*.

- **Type III.** This is a more severe level of widening of the part and more diffuse thinning over the top of the scalp. Thankfully, this more devastating type of hair loss is less common, occurring in only 5 percent of women.

Ludwig Classification Scale

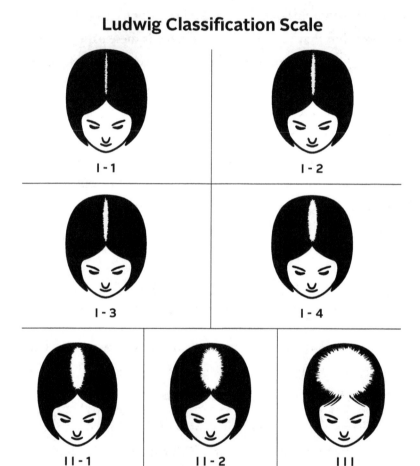

While the Ludwig is the more commonly used scale in determining a woman's level of hair loss in clinical practice, there are a few other classification scales used largely for research studies and dermatology.[19] These include the following:

- **Ebling and Rook**. This is a five-stage classification scale with the first three stages mirroring the Ludwig scale.

- **Savin.** This is an eight-stage classification scale that shows more thinning at the crown.

- **Olsen.** This is a three-stage classification scale that has a more defined triangle-shaped loss.

- **Gan-Sinclair Scale.** This is a five-stage classification scale that involves a patient self-identifying their degree of loss.

While these scales are helpful for clinicians in diagnosing hair thinning and loss, the bottom line is that most patients don't really care what stage of XYZ classification they're in. They just want to know, "Doctor, what can you do to help me get my hair back?"

MEDICAL OR PROCEDURAL TREATMENTS

As with men, in females we start by looking at some of the medical and procedural treatments that may work for the patient. Some of the same medical treatment options that we discussed for men also work for women, but there are differences—some significant—in their usage.

---

19 M. Gupta and V. Mysore, "Classifications of Patterned Hair Loss: A Review," *Journal of Cutaneous and Aesthetic Surgery*, vol. 9, issue 1 (2016), 3–12, doi:10.4103/0974-2077.178536.

THE TRUTH ABOUT HAIR RESTORATION

MYTH: Hair restoration options are only designed to work on men.

TRUTH: There are many options for women, including medical, procedural, and surgical.

Minoxidil. This works in maybe 30 percent of women and takes at least a couple of months to see results. It must be used long term to maintain the results. Most patients tolerate it well, with dry scalp or itching being the main side effects. However, it should be applied only where hair growth is desired because it will create growth wherever it's applied.

Rogaine is the most common brand name for minoxidil, which is a vasodilator, meaning it helps increase blood flow to the scalp wherever it's applied. It helps some of the small hairs grow stronger and thicker, giving the appearance of some regrowth. Minoxidil increases the duration of the growth phase of the hair cycle, so you tend to get more thicker hair and less miniaturized hair growing for a longer period of time.

With women, we typically prescribe a 5 percent solution, which is available where I practice only as a prescription. Some practices only recommend the 2 percent version because it is available over the counter.

Spironolactone. Spironolactone is a medication that's only available for women. Men can't take it because it is an anti-androgen, meaning it will negatively affect a man's hormones.

It's especially helpful for women who have polycystic ovarian syndrome (PCOS), which causes significant excess of androgen or male hormones. That excess androgen can cause a woman to have a lot of acne, hair growth in unwanted areas, and hair loss where they want it, up on the scalp.

Women who take spironolactone typically are also placed on an oral contraceptive because there is the potential for congenital abnormalities to form, especially in a male fetus, should a woman become pregnant while taking it. It should not be prescribed to women who are considering getting pregnant, and extra precautions should be taken to avoid pregnancy.

Side effects with spironolactone include weight gain, loss of libido, depression, and fatigue.

Finasteride. We usually reserve finasteride as an option for post-menopausal women. Topical and oral options are available, and it is available as a compound through some pharmacies.

Biotin, vitamins, and supplements. Especially for women who have diffused hair, we encourage taking biotin, a coenzyme that helps the function of B-complex vitamins, along with vitamins A, B complex, C, D, and E and the minerals zinc, iodine, and iron.

Nutrafol. This is a commercially available product that is available for men, but also in a special formulation for women. Nutrafol is marketed as a Synergen complex, which includes ingredients such as a very potent form of vitamin E; ashwagandha, an Indian ginseng known as a stress and anxiety reducer; saw palmetto, a natural DHT blocker; curcumin, a powerful antioxidant; and marine collagen, for healthier skin. The women's version also has maca root and other anti-inflammatories that have been shown to be effective.

Low Laser Light Therapy (LLLT)

Low laser light therapy (LLLT), also known as a laser cap, is a very good option for women. This can be an especially good option when a woman is not a good candidate for hair transplantation.

As I mentioned in chapter 3, lasers are a specialized kind of light that target chromophores in tissue, which include melanin, a pigment in the skin and hair follicles, hemoglobin in blood, and water within the tissue.

LLLT is a less invasive option that can be very helpful for any type of hair loss because it can reverse miniaturization and slow thinning. It can thicken the hairs that are not thinning, making the hair appear fuller and denser. Laser caps are very low risk and tolerated really well, and treatment can easily be done at home. It doesn't take long before the treatment becomes a habit. I had a mother-daughter pair of patients who suffered from a genetic type of diffused hair loss who shared a laser cap, since the treatment only takes about six minutes a day. The treatment worked very well for both of them.

The lasers target the hair follicles, which are only five or six millimeters into the scalp. The treatment works, it's theorized, because the lasers make the follicles happy by stimulating circulation and oxygenation, causing them to shift into the growing phase. That allows the miniaturized hairs to stay in the growing phase longer and then rest for a shorter period of time, giving the appearance of much more hair and more coverage.

Platelet-Rich Plasma (PRP) Treatments

Platelet-rich plasma (PRP) treatments are also a viable option for women, primarily for those with miniaturization that may be reversible.

To recap some of the lengthier discussion from chapter 3, PRP treatments involve spinning down your whole blood to concentrate the platelets and release their growth factors. These growth factors stimulate stem cells, which help with wound healing, and can stimulate hair follicle growth and the formation of new blood vessels.

You may have heard of PRP because it is being used for everything from facial plastic surgery to dentistry. But it's also proving to be a viable option for many patients for the treatment of various types of alopecia, especially androgenic alopecia—it's a little like fertilizer for the hair follicles. Since it involves using your own blood, it is a very safe treatment option.

Please refer back to chapter 3 for more information on PRP studies and results, and more about the treatment process itself.

As with other treatments, before we look at PRP as a treatment, we do a lab workup and scalp biopsy to try to figure out the cause of the hair loss. For many women, PRP can be very effective, especially in combination with some of these other treatments.

HAIR TRANSPLANTATION

To be a candidate for hair transplantation—and this goes for men and women, but especially women—there really has to be a stable donor area. Regardless of the cause or degree of hair loss, a stable donor area—hair along the back and sides of the scalp—is the key criterion. That can be especially difficult if a woman has

To be a candidate for hair transplantation—and this goes for men and women, but especially women—there really has to be a stable donor area.

diffused female pattern loss and there is miniaturization in the back of the scalp. If miniaturization is already prominent in the donor areas, we don't want to take the hairs out and transplant them up top, because they will not successfully live there permanently like they did in the donor area where they were located.

So we are very cautious when it comes to hair transplants for women. Often, before we'll consider transplantation, we'll recommend following the patient for at least a year to see how they're responding to other treatments. We'll watch their progression and rule out different causes based on the lab tests and biopsy results. And we want to make sure that they have a very stable donor area before we even consider a transplantation.

Before we determine that a transplant is a viable option, we have to first determine whether a patient is a viable candidate.

> *As a woman, it was unnatural to have a receding hairline. I felt like I looked unhealthy and older than I am. I did not have an extreme situation, but a nagging discomfort. I thought a procedure of any kind would be extreme until I looked into what Dr. Angelos is doing. I took a leap of faith, and it was the most effortless and successful experience. Dr. Angelos is a skilled surgeon and an artist. In hindsight, I cannot believe I was ever on the fence.* **—Patient**

Good Candidates for Transplant

According to the American Hair Loss Association, only 2 to 5 percent of women are actually good candidates for hair transplantation. Here are some of the factors that help determine candidacy:

Mechanical or traction alopecia. Women with mechanical or traction alopecia are typically good candidates for transplant. Again, this is very localized hair loss that occurs typically as a result of wearing very tight braids, dreadlocks, or weaves. If the hair loss does not respond well to medical or procedural treatments, then transplantation may be an option, as long as there is donor hair available.

Previous scalp surgery. Previous scalp surgery that has left alopecia around the scar may make a woman a good candidate for transplantation. That scarring may be the result of plastic surgery procedures, such as some of the facelift procedures that require incisions in the scalp. Transplantation can help fill in density around those scars.

Trauma and burns. Sutures from traumatic injuries and severe burns can cause scarring in the scalp. Again, transplantation may be a good option to fill in those areas where hair no longer grows.

Male pattern baldness in a female. As long as there is a very stable donor area with normal density and all that's needed is a little filler up front in the temporal recession areas or the crown, then a woman with the familiar male pattern baldness may be an ideal candidate for transplantation.

Alopecia marginalis. Although rarer, alopecia marginalis is similar to traction alopecia, but it is more of a hereditary condition that results in loss at the front of the hairline and the temples.

Less-Than-Ideal Candidates

There are a couple of key reasons a woman might not be an ideal candidate for hair transplantation.

Diffused thinning in the donor area. Earlier, I mentioned the different types of hair loss in women. Transplantation is not an option for those who have completely diffused thinning that includes the donor area.

Unrealistic expectations. Another reason a woman might not be a good candidate for transplantation is unrealistic expectations. For instance, transplantation might be able to increase hair density for someone who has moderately diffused thinning in the front and on top, but it may not give them a full head of hair like they had previously.

If a female patient has a widening part that is very localized, she wears her hair a certain way, and the hair loss has been stable for many years, then we want to rule out causes to ensure that the donor area truly is stable and that the results of a transplant can produce some realistic expectations. Typically, on average, less than 20 percent of the donor area should have miniaturization for the goals of transplantation to be realistic.

We then determine whether we can transplant from the donor area to help fill in density and help them wear their hair that certain style.

Especially when it comes to hair transplantation in women, surgeons need to be very realistic about the results. It's true in men as well as women, but in my practice, we spend a little more time discussing expectations with women because they often want full density like they had when they were a teenager. Unfortunately, that's often not possible, especially in women with more advanced hair loss. With transplantation, we're not increasing the hair follicle count in the scalp. We're just redistributing what's already there—we're moving hair from one area where there is more hair to another area where there is less hair.

The bottom line is that if there are one or two areas that are noticeable, good results can be achieved, and the patient's goals and expectations merge with what the surgeon thinks they can deliver, then transplantation may be a good option. Even posttransplant, the results may limit the hairstyles you can wear because the procedure itself may cause some thinning in an area, and you will need to style your hair so that the area is not exposed. For women, it may come down to deciding which part line is most important, how you want to wear your hair, and how we can best help you with redistributing some of the hair through transplantation.

The areas we commonly transplant in women include the hairline; just behind the hairline; temporal recession areas, especially in male pattern loss in a female; along the part line; and sometimes the crown.

However, these days, we can even transplant hairs into eyebrows and eyelashes.

Eyebrows and Eyelashes

Over time, eyebrows have trended from full and bushy to very thin. With the latter of these, women may wax and pluck their brows to the point of having thinning and hair loss. Aging eyebrows sometimes also have significant thinning.

To remedy the situation, women often use makeup to fill in gaps or fill out their brows, while others resort to having eyebrows tattooed back on.

A more natural-looking result, however, involves transplantation.

With both eyebrow and eyelash transplantation, the transplanted hair may require additional grooming, depending on where it is harvested from. If it is harvested from the back of the scalp, just like we do with most hair transplants, then the hair will grow as long as it would on the scalp. Body hair does not grow as fast or as long, so there is less grooming needed when body hair is transplanted to the eyebrows or eyelashes. Although earlier in the book I mentioned how transplanted hair does tend to adapt to its new home, it will not adapt completely in the eyebrows and eyelashes. Salons offer lash lifts and perms for eyelashes since transplanted hairs don't have a natural curl like normal eyelashes do.

DESIGNING THE HARVEST AREA AND HAIRLINE—THERE'S AN ART TO IT

The FUE procedure involves shaving the hair in the donor area, something women are especially not eager to do. But with women, the good news is that we can pull up their longer hair, create a harvest site, and then lay their hair back down over the site. That way the harvest area is rarely visible. The ARTAS robotic hair restoration system lets us work around the long hair at the implant site, so there's no need to shave anywhere except that small harvest site under the long hair in the back of the scalp.

Again, we want to be sure that the donor area is stable, with ideally less than 20 percent miniaturizing, so we use a densitometer to ensure that we're leaving enough hair behind, and that the hairs being harvested and transplanted will not fall out later.

It's especially important to have an accurate diagnosis with women, particularly those who are younger, because later hair loss could involve the donor area and transplanted hairs may eventually fall out. Where hair transplantation is essentially permanent in men, it's more of a relative permanence in women if the donor area is not truly safe and is in the process of miniaturization. That's why a good portion of women are really not good candidates for transplant.

Don't get me wrong: it can be very rewarding for a woman to undergo a successful hair transplant. Especially when there is male pattern loss in a female, transplantation can make a big difference. That's far and away the most common scenario we see in female patients. They come in and tell us that male pattern baldness runs in their family, and that the other women in their family have the same pattern of hair loss. Once we take labs and a scalp biopsy, if we feel like they've been stable on some medical treatments and the donor area has really good density, then we've found that they can get a really nice result with transplanting.

But when some of the other causes are evident, and the loss is more diffused, then they can still get some good results with medical and procedural treatments such as laser caps and PRP.

When "designing" a hair line, some providers want to look at the hair when it's wet and again when it is dry to get a feel what the patient would benefit from most. I tend to agree with Dr. Robin Unger of New York, who says transplantation is about creating "the illusion of density with the fewest number of hairs," and that it is easiest to see when the hair is dry.[20]

In chapter 8, I share more about some of the factors to look for in a hair restoration specialist. But first, let's look at some of the exciting emerging technologies that may be available in the years to come.

---

20   Unger, et al., *Hair Transplantation*.

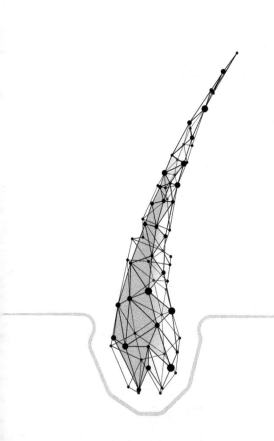

CHAPTER 7

EMERGING TECHNOLOGIES

*T*he future is exciting with all that's on the horizon for hair restoration. I'm especially excited about the idea of gene therapy and regenerative medicine in general, but see some really interesting potential for them in hair restoration. Certainly, it would be great if we could find a cure, a way to prevent hair loss from the start. That would be the biggest breakthrough.

But we're not there yet. Here are some of the advances as I write this book.

BETTER MEDICATIONS

One of the trends that we're already seeing in medications are more topical DHT blockers, including finasteride, sold under the brand name Propecia, which is an oral tablet. One of the downsides of taking finasteride orally is that it has systemic or full body side effects. For that reason, surgeons are starting to move more toward using compounding pharmacies to formulate topical DHT blockers to avoid those side effects.

Research into hair loss is also starting to target the "bulge" or middle part of the hair follicle where cells are that are believed to be responsible for regrowing the follicle at the beginning of a new growth phase of the cycle. That may be a target to prevent hair loss in general with potentially a new therapeutic drug or a technique or procedure that keeps those cells continuing to grow instead of dying off.

Research is also looking at ways to induce hair cells to be less sensitive to DHT, a male hormone in the body that is one of the factors contributing to hair thinning and loss. As I've explained, the donor area on the back and sides of the scalp are resistant to DHT. Through gene therapy or medication, it may one day be possible to make the top of the scalp resistant to DHT, even with a genetic predisposition.

FUTURE SURGICAL TREATMENTS

Some of the advances in surgical treatments are more near term and essentially extensions of what we're already doing in robotics and AI technology. For instance, the maker of ARTAS, which is already leading the robotics transplantation industry, is working on advances that will increase the speed, accuracy, and precision of the system. Harvest times will be shorter, and the efficiency of the harvest process will improve. As AI technology gets

> The maker of ARTAS, which is already leading the robotics transplantation industry, is working on advances that will increase the speed, accuracy, and precision of the system.

smarter, it will be better at selecting grafts—it will be more personalized to each case and the needs of each patient. At some point, the ARTAS may eliminate some of the need for human hair techs as well. While it may never be a fully robotic procedure, requiring at least some supervision, the company is working on advances to make the process more streamlined and more automated, and to as much as possible reduce the amount of human manpower and time and energy needed.

STEM CELL TREATMENT: THE BASICS

There are several types of stem cells that function differently and therefore have different capabilities. To help you understand them better, let me explain some of the terms involved in stem cell treatments and regenerative medicine.

THE TRUTH ABOUT HAIR RESTORATION

MYTH: As men age, the quantity of stem cells in the scalp diminish.

TRUTH: Bald men have the same number of stem cells in their scalps as do men with full heads of hair.

Pluripotent. Pluripotent cells can essentially be turned into any type of cell in the body except for germ cells (which determine male or female sex).

Embryonic stem cells. You've likely already heard about embryonic stem cells, the cells in an embryo that are pluripotent. These days, embryonic stem cells are available commercially in some areas to be used by researchers or in experimental clinical situations.

Adult stem cells. Adult stem cells are typically taken from fat, bone marrow, or blood. Adult stem cells are multipotent, meaning they have limited lines of cells that they can turn into. For example, stem cells from blood may be able to turn into different types of cells, but not just any type of cell—they do not have the same potential as embryonic cells. Adult stem cells are already being used in certain areas of medicine to help with healing, et cetera, but currently, they are not widely used in hair transplantation, except anecdotally and experimentally.

Autologous. Most of the stem cell treatments for hair transplantation are autologous. That means the treatment uses the person's own stem cells harvested from their own bone marrow, blood, or fat. Researchers have already discovered that stem cells can also be harvested from the bulge part of the follicle, making it possible to harvest a person's cells.

The future of hair restoration will include regenerative medicine with stem cell cloning, hair multiplication, and gene therapy.

HAIR CLONING

Ultimately, through propagation and hair cloning, the hope is that research will develop the ability to have a limitless supply of hair without sacrificing a large amount of donor hair. To do that, one of the goals is to develop ways to grow hair in the lab. In clinical application, that might mean harvesting a small sample of hair out of the back of someone's scalp and using it to grow a limitless number of grafts to implant back into the scalp. That would eliminate concerns about depleting the donor supply, which can happen during an aggressive hair transplant surgery in the hands of some techs.

To better understand cloning, let's look briefly at how human hair grows.

The hair begins to grow from the root or follicle. As it develops, it pushes up the hair shaft above it. In some places on the body, it stops once it reaches a certain length. The hair on top of the head and in the beard continue to grow indefinitely, though that growth may slow down over time.

In order to grow, the hair needs several "ingredients," including the following:

- Protein cells to create the hair itself

- Blood to feed the root, bringing it oxygen and nutrients

- Oil to keep the hair shiny, soft, pliable, and safe from breakage

- Chemical stimulants, called growth factors, to tell hair to continue growing from the follicle

- Productive follicles

There is evidence that stem cells may help by retriggering the growth and reproduction of cells in an area of the body that was formerly too old or damaged to do so on its own—for example, dying off hair follicles that have stopped producing normal hair. As I've explained, hair loss is progressive, and hairs miniaturize until the follicle stops producing hair. But that follicle itself may not be totally "dead," so to speak, and it can essentially be reawakened by stem cells to start growing again.

That's a really attractive target in regenerative medicine because hair follicles are a very specialized skin structure that are not exceedingly simple, but not exceedingly complex either. Using stem cells to regenerate follicles is not like making a heart or other vital organ, which are clearly much more complicated.

THE PROGRESSION OF RESEARCH

Let's look at what's been done in regenerative research and what the future holds.

In 1993, researchers Jahoda and Reynolds had the first success at growing a rat whisker in a live rat from cultured rat dermal papilla cells.[21] A year later, in 1994, the same group was able to grow what was essentially the first test tube hair.

Hair Multiplication

Only a few years later, in 1998, Dr. Gho of the Hair Science Institute in the Netherlands patented with the World Intellectual Property Organization, a "method for the propagation of hair" in which he described a method of plucking hairs in the anagen (growth) phase, and culturing the dermal papilla cells from the portion of the hair bulb at the end of the plucked hair. He described using commercial cell culture media along with various beneficial additives such as amino acids, vitamins, trace elements, growth hormones, and antibiotics. His patent seems to imply that the best results are achieved by also adding cloned CD34+ progenitor cells, a type of stem cell, to the culture.

His process, known as hair multiplication, involved harvesting a hair follicle, splitting it in half, placing one of the halves back into

---

21   Colin A. B. Jahoda, Amanda J. Reynolds, and Roy F. Oliver, "Induction of Hair Growth in Ear Wounds by Cultured Dermal Papilla Cells," *Journal of Investigative Dermatology* vol. 101, issue 4 (October 1993), 584-90.

the scalp, and then using the other half in the lab to generate more hairs. One half was placed back into the scalp to avoid decreasing donor density and to allow the hair follicle to produce another hair in the scalp. Since the half at the lab contained some fat and blood, stem cells could be isolated from that half of the follicle and used to stimulate and duplicate hair follicles in the lab. The process did not necessarily provide an unlimited supply like cloning might, but it could produce many hairs. The donor follicles with the stem cells were then injected back into the scalp to stimulate regrowth and could even signal some of the other follicles already there that were not producing hair to restart making hair as well.

Clinically, the procedure is ongoing in the Netherlands, ranging in price from $3,000 to $10,000 per treatment, with patients doing one to six treatments total.

RepliCel's Cell Therapy. RepliCel is a Vancouver, British Columbia, biotech company that is developing an autologous cell therapy utilizing dermal sheath cup (DSC) cells, isolated from punch biopsies, to treat androgenic alopecia. This process is similar to the hair multiplication therapy in the Netherlands, where the cells are multiplied in the lab and injected back into balding areas on the patient's scalp. The treatment, known as RCH-01, is now under clinical investigation at the Tokyo Medical University Hospital and Toho University Ohasi Medical Center in Japan. Phase II of the clinical trial has been completed; however there appears to be a licensing dispute between RepliCel and Shiseido, a Japanese personal care company, that is holding up commercialization of RCH-01. Here again, the goal with RCH-01 is to immunize hair follicles prone to DHT sensitivity.

THE 3-D "SCAFFOLDS" RACE

One of the biggest challenges in achieving consistent results with growing stem cell hair is retaining the shape of the bulb. The problem is that it's difficult to get dermal papilla cells to self-aggregate into a teardrop shape for the hair follicle. Instead of automatically shaping themselves, the cells tend to spread out in the culture and then revert back to basic skin cells. Because hair cells are really a specialized part of the skin-type cell, when they're not in that physical three-dimensional organization of a bulb or a teardrop-shaped follicle, they don't continue to act like hair. They start to act more like skin.

A big discovery to overcome the problem came by creating 3-D "scaffolds" that mimic the shape of a hair bulb. There has been a considerable amount of research into a biodegradable scaffold that the hair matrix can be grown in; instead of a flat petri dish, the cells are placed in a scaffold that literally looks like a hair follicle bulb. By shaping the cells into the correct orientation, they are able to grow into true hair. The result is, more or less, a limitless supply of hair follicles to use in transplantation; instead of having only three thousand to work with, now there might be ten thousand.

The discovery that hair stem cells need to stay aggregated in their teardrop shape to continue to grow and signal growth has launched a global "arms race" to generate sustainable hair follicles that will hold their shape.

Stemson Therapeutics, a San Diego–based start-up, is working on cloning hair follicles. The company is growing hair from stem cells derived from a person's own skin or blood, and then implanting hair follicles rich with dermal papillae into the space around a person's old, shrunken, dormant follicles.

According to the International Society for Stem Cell Research, human hair follicles have been successfully transplanted into mice.[22] At the society's annual meeting, the CEO, Geoff Hamilton, proposed one solution involving a synthetic scaffold, which he claims is proprietary. The scaffold would be implanted around the cloned follicle to direct the growth of the hair. Stemson Therapeutics partnered with the pharmaceutical giant Allergan to develop this scaffold for cloned hair, and as I write this, trials are expected to start soon.

Meanwhile, Angela Christiano, a professor of genetics and dermatology at Columbia University, has used 3-D printing to generate a gelatin mold that holds the follicle and dermal papillae in place as they differentiate into hair. She reported the results in the journal *Nature Communications*, stating that the ability to regenerate an entire hair from cultured human cells "will have a transformative impact on the medical management of different types of alopecia, as well as chronic wounds."[23] This new technique is a huge landmark.

The challenge remains as to what happens if that scaffold biodegrades: Does the cloned hair follicle continue to hold its shape and act like a hair? Does it eventually differentiate back into a normal skin cell and stop producing hair? Will it grow indefinitely without constantly needing more stem cells being pumped in to signal the molecules to keep growing?

Another potential concern is that these cloned hairs may only grow for their first cycle. They'll go through their anagen, catagen,

---

22 Hasan Erbil Abaci, Abigail Coffman, Yanne Doucet, James Chen, Joanna Jacków, Etienne Wang, Zongyou Guo, Jung U. Shin, Colin A. Jahoda, and Angela M. Christiano. "Tissue engineering of human hair follicles using a biomimetic developmental approach," *Nature Communications*, vol. 9, article 5301 (December 13, 2018). doi:10.1038/s41467-018-07579-y.

23 Hasan Erbil Abaci, Abigail Coffman, Yanne Doucet, James Chen, Joanna Jacków, Etienne Wang, Zongyou Guo, Jung U. Shin, Colin A. Jahoda, and Angela M. Christiano. "Tissue engineering of human hair follicles using a biomimetic developmental approach," *Nature Communications*, vol. 9, article 5301 (December 13, 2018). doi:10.1038/s41467-018-07579-y.

and telogen phases, but then may stop. They may not continue to cycle like the natural hairs on the scalp that are living indefinitely.

Other challenges include difficulty generating normal hairs and follicles—in other words, hair quality: correct color, texture, angulation, and direction. Again, that's being improved with scaffolds, but the results may still not be perfect and aesthetically pleasing.

A general consensus right now is that, early on at least, cloned hair may be used more as filler after hair transplantation surgery to create more density. It could be especially useful if someone is out of donor hair. But on its own, cloned hair still has a way to go before it is the end-all solution for transplantation.

Other obstacles that may delay advances include dealing with FDA regulations and requirements. That can take many years, but it's obviously essential for patient safety. Then there are also some long-term theoretical safety risks with stem cell treatments. Unlike other transplants, hair transplantation is not something that can be done from another source, for instance, from another person. But when the stem cells are not in their original location, there may be concerns about them potentially forming tumors or even multiplying and migrating to the other areas of the body. For example, skin cancers might be a potential concern. There is certainly some concern about patients who have autoimmune conditions and how stem cell therapies may affect the way the immune system functions in an area of the body. Basically, there may be some unintended consequences that won't really be understood until some of these things are studied in the long term.

Still, I'm really excited about these technologies and their use in hair restoration. Yes, there are challenges and hurdles to overcome. Like any new technology in the field, in my practice, we like to see the experimental evidence, use in clinical practice, and the long-term effectiveness before we start trying this on our own patients. We definitely want to make sure that it's safe and effective long term.

At least early on, the cost for these treatments will likely be tremendous. But I believe that as these come to the forefront and become more tried and true, we will be able to partner with a regenerative medicine-type lab and be able to offer them to our patients.

Now, let's look at some of the factors to look for in a hair restoration specialist.

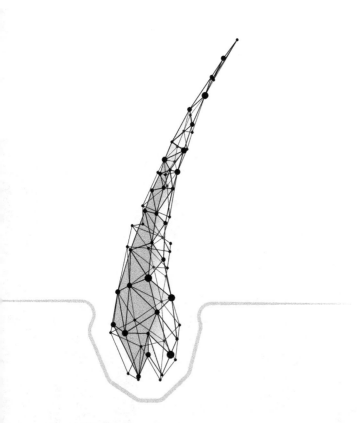

CHAPTER 8

WHAT TO LOOK FOR IN A HAIR
RESTORATION SPECIALIST

*A*s the Southeast's leader in the latest hair restoration technology, my skilled team and I deliver the most appropriate solutions for hair thinning and loss. Whether it's a medical or procedural treatment, an FUE or other surgery, or a robotic solution using the ARTAS iX, we offer a full set of options to address specific needs and do what's best for each patient.

But every provider is different, and you'll want to find the one that you trust for your hair restoration needs. So how do you that? Here are some factors to consider when identifying the best provider for you.

Board certification. Look for core aesthetic specialties like dermatology, plastic surgery, facial plastic surgery, and otolaryngology/head-and-neck surgery. All of these have rigorous standards of training and certification, including maintenance of certification (MOC). In my opinion, these are the most qualified types of medical providers to evaluate and treat hair loss to and to perform hair transplantation surgery. That doesn't mean that other types of doctors can't do hair transplantation and hair restoration, but these core specialties are the ones that have been specifically trained in it.

Doctors may also be recognized by the American Board of Hair Restoration Surgery (ABHRS) and the International Society of Hair Restoration Surgery (ISHRS). If a provider does not have the core specialties that I mentioned, then look for membership or certification in one or both of these societies.

A comprehensive consultation. How much time does the doctor spend in the consultation, especially answering questions and concerns? Does the doctor take enough time to do a thorough history, exam, and assessment up front? Are the recommendations specific to your needs, not just an automatic recommendation for surgery because it's the only treatment offered? Unfortunately, that happens in some hair transplantation practices—make sure you don't feel too pressured to undergo surgery and that you're given the opportunity to ask questions and understand all of your options.

> Make sure you don't feel too pressured to undergo surgery and that you're given the opportunity to ask questions and understand all of your options.

In my practice, patients meet with both the physician (me) and the nurse, who acts as the consultant. We find that meeting directly with the providers promotes more consistent results from start to finish. We take about an hour to discuss your specific situation, and then often answer calls afterward or set up a second consultation.

We try to be very candid with patients. We want them to understand the factors they have going for them, and some that may make treatment somewhat limited. We want patients to know if they do not have the best donor area or their hair loss is advanced enough that they need to be realistic about their goals.

We also want them to understand what other options may be best for them without overselling or rushing them to a decision.

Full set of options. Does the provider offer medical, procedural, and surgical solutions, including robotic transplantation? What methods of hair transplantation does the practice offer and what technologies? Instead of only robotics, look for a provider that offers a full set of options so that the solution can be tailored to your needs.

Years of experience. How long has the provider been in practice? I started residency in 2006 and have been performing surgery on patients ever since.

Percentage of practice solely dedicated to hair transplantation. Look for a provider who is consistently performing hair restoration as part of their practice, not just occasionally or rarely. Hair restoration does not need to be their only service, but it should be a significant portion of their practice, where they're seeing hair restoration patients a minimum of 25 percent of the time.

Type of anesthesia. What type of anesthesia do you use? And who administers and monitors the anesthesia? As the physician, I administer and monitor any anesthesia used in procedures and surgeries. It's not done by an assistant or technician.

A dedicated team. Often, when providers are just starting to offer restoration and have not completed many cases, they will bring in contractors to help perform the procedure. They don't really have a consistent team, which can lead to inconsistent results.

Look for a provider whose team members are employed by the practice and ideally who have been trained by the surgeon. You want a team that communicates and works well together to help you reach your goals.

At the Hair Restoration Center, we have a very consistent team, including an internally trained technician, an on-staff nurse, and me, the surgeon.

"Bedside manner" matters. Any type of surgery can be an uneasy experience, physically and mentally, and hair restoration is no different. That's why you want a highly professional, caring team that takes the time to educate and inform, and to alleviate your fears and anxieties. You want someone that you can trust to help you have the outcome you desire.

Follow-up to help lifelong goals fit in with short-term goals. One of the big challenges that's recognized in hair restoration is that patients tend to come in with short-term goals. They want to get back a full head of hair before a wedding or anniversary or reunion—next year. It's up to the physician to guide the patient through big-picture goals. For instance, plans for a thirty-one-year-old with significantly progressive hair loss problem should not only include having hair for their wedding next year, but also making sure that the patient is on some kind of longer-term treatment regimen and is aware that another hair transplant procedure may be down the road. Because focusing only on the short-term goal of filling in hair for a wedding may then result in hair that looks inappropriate in another ten years when more hair is lost.

At the Hair Restoration Center, we put together a master plan that fits both short- and long-term goals. We want you to have the best-looking hair that's appropriate to you throughout all the ages of your life.

Artistry and the quality. Granted, hair transplantation is not rocket surgery. The procedures can actually be performed by people with very little training and no specific credentialing, so it has become an add-on procedure for some providers who are not schooled or skilled at procedural medicine.

It's the artistry that sets providers apart. That's where training as a plastic surgeon really makes a difference—artistically restoring the body is something that we plastic surgeons do every day.

Hair restoration is a time-consuming process—it can even be a tedious process for the provider. The last thing you want is a provider who tires during your procedure and rushes just to finish the work.

Look for a doctor and team who love what they do, who have a lifelong interest in science, art, and medicine. Your provider should care about your results as much as you do.

Patient results. Ask about before-and-after results. Does the practice have photos of its patients? Are there patients whom you can talk to about their experience with the doctor, the team, and the procedure?

Dr. Angelos is amazing! I couldn't be happier with my results. I will continue to see him. Super friendly and very easy to talk to. I highly recommend him! **—Ambra**

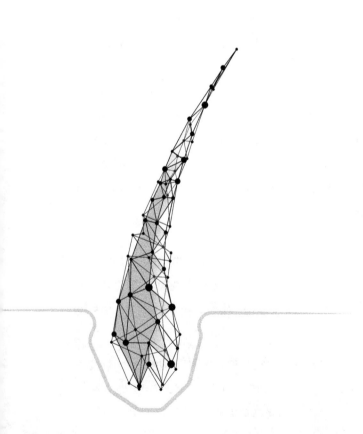

CONCLUSION

*T*oo often, people put off hair restoration treatment because there is so much information—or misinformation—about what works, and what doesn't. With so many solutions available today, gone are the days of "doll's hair" restorations—those little plugs that just don't look like natural hair. And the options that we have today are for both men and women. They are very natural looking and not terribly rigorous, so they make for a much better experience, and much better results.

I hope by what I've shared in this book, you have a much clearer picture of why hair loss occurs and some of the options available today for restoring hair. For both men and women, there are medical, procedural, and surgical options depending on the causes of—and the potential for future—thinning and hair loss.

Remember, medical options include both topical and oral treatments that produce some very good results when used consistently. Consistency is also key to success with some of the nonsurgical treatments, such as low laser light therapy (LLLT), also known as a laser cap, and platelet-rich plasma (PRP), which is derived from your own blood.

And then there are surgical options, which I've explained. Some of the most viable of these involve follicular unit extraction (FUE), a tried-and-true method for creating very natural-looking results.

Today, those results are even more pleasing, thanks to the state-of-the-art ARTAS robotics restoration system. My practice, the Hair Restoration Center at Charleston Plastic Surgery, was the first in the state to have this technology, and we decided to add it to our hair restoration tool kit after realizing there was no one else in the area that we felt comfortable referring patients to. It's been a welcome addition that has been giving patients some life-changing results.

But remember: While hair transplantation is ideal for some types of hair loss, it is not the solution for everyone in every situation. If that's the only solution a provider offers, consider looking elsewhere, because what's most important is that *any solution may be right for you and your specific type of hair loss.*

While the causes of hair loss in men are most often attributed to the same basic factors—aging, heredity, and stress—that does not mean everyone should be a candidate for the same treatment. We also know that hair loss is particularly devastating for women, yet treatment must be even more specialized because of women's specific situations.

That's why we create individualized treatment plans that are designed to meet your short-term and long-term goals. We know that restoring hair with an eye on future hair loss will bring you the most satisfying, superior results.

What it all boils down to is understanding your options. By reading this book, you've taken the first step in educating yourself about some of the potential reasons behind your hair loss, and some of the treatments that might be options for you.

Whether you're a man in your twenties and just beginning to notice some thinning, a man in your sixties experiencing advanced hair loss, or a woman distressed by areas where your scalp is beginning to show, I hope you are now equipped with some basic information to help you better understand your options and what to look for in a provider.

If that provider is the Hair Restoration Center at Charleston Plastic Surgery, then your experience will be one that combines both science and art to give you the best short- and long-term results. We take a caring and compassionate approach to hair restoration—we want to first understand you and your situation and then look at solutions that can begin to produce results today that will still look natural in the years to come as your situation continues to change.

I love what I do. I love seeing patients' confidence levels change during our initial consult and then as treatment progresses. It's very exciting to see the treatments we offer produce some very life-changing results.

With all the advances we have available today for hair restoration, there's no better time to seek out a provider for a consult and discover the options best suited to you.

If you'd like to know more, reach out to us at the Hair Restoration Center at Charleston Plastic Surgery.

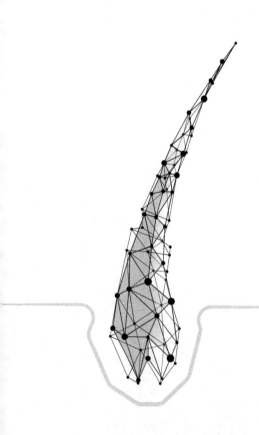

OUR SERVICES

THE HAIR RESTORATION CENTER at Charleston Plastic Surgery offers a full set of options for hair restoration, including medical and procedural, nonsurgical, and surgical. These include:

- Topical treatments—Rogaine (minoxidil)

- Oral medications—Propecia, Nutrafol

- Capillus laser light therapy

- Platelet-rich plasma therapy

- Surgical treatments

- ARTAS robotics hair transplantation

For more information or to schedule a consultation, please visit us:

The Hair Restoration Center at Charleston Plastic Surgery Center

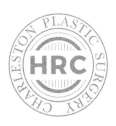

2295 Henry Tecklenburg Drive
Charleston, South Carolina 29414
Phone: 843-882-HAIR
https://chashairrestoration.com
https://drpatrickangelos.com

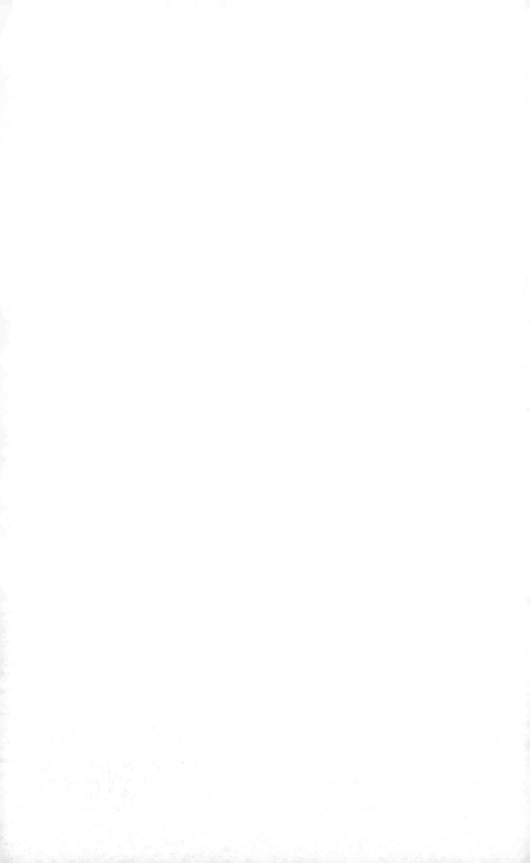